Managing Incontinence

Cheryle Gartley, Editor

Jameson Books
Ottawa, Illinois

Jameson Books, Inc.
722 Columbus St.
Ottawa, IL 61350

(815) 434-7905

Jameson books are available at special discounts for bulk purchases for sales promotions, premiums, fund-raising, or educational use. Special editions can also be created to specification. For details contact Special Sales Director, Jameson Books, P.O. Box 738, Ottawa, IL 61350.

10   9   8   7   6   5   4

Printed in the United States of America

Contents

Preface

Freedom is a rich and wonderful gift; delicious, intoxicating, so easy to take for granted, until it is gone.

Cheryle Gartley has never accepted the theft of her freedom, the confinement incontinence has imposed on her and on so many other people. Live with it yes, tolerate it no. She is angry and frustrated, but she is not willing to wrap herself in embarrassment and hide, and she is not willing to be silent.

Incontinence is something you're not suppose to talk about, but it's time someone did start talking, started shouting, crying for action from the society that has unconsciously put thousands of Cheryle Gartleys under house arrest.

Incontinence is for women an even bigger problem than for men, because there is no device, no collection tube manufactured that really fits a woman's body. So where are the women's groups whose crusading has forced recognition of rape and breast cancer and incest as important legitimate issues to be confronted and dealt with openly?

If we can talk about impotence, why not incontinence?

Yesterday's taboos have become today's soap operas, daytime television dramas. But when was the last time you saw this on afternoon television—a luscious young woman sobbing, her fiancé, disgusted by her incontinence problem and scornful of her, having walked out? Or this—a smooth, megabucks manipulator excusing himself in a low voice, and rushing suddenly from a key meeting, leaving his board of directors stunned, whispering among themselves?

You think I'm joking. I'm not. These are scenes of painful personal crisis, as real and emotional as any others. If people watch television characters they empathize with who are coping with controversial problems, they are willing to learn. Ten years ago rape and child abuse and alcoholism had not yet become acceptable television tragedies either. Now look.

Bang bang is great for television news—Beirut, Central America—the bloodier the better. I know. I've been there. But when I did a gentle, discreetly crafted piece showing a baby being born I was told childbirth was sickening to watch on television, distasteful, unsuitable for a news program.

5

The piece never ran. Not long before, the same broadcast had given prominent coverage to a crowd of poor Indians being machine-gunned on the steps of the cathedral in San Salvador, their bodies twitching as they died. This is the priority system that determines incontinence is not a subject for mass media.

Barriers fall slowly, but they do fall. With awareness comes change. A few talk shows have "discovered" incontinence, but it is not enough just to tell the public the problem exists. Someone has to teach people who are incontinent to talk to each other, to put aside shame, to step out of the shadowy netherworld they never knew they shared, to identify themselves, and to demand help; then together to knock on the doors of research institutions and medical products manufacturers until someone answers.

I believe that Cheryle Gartley is articulate enough and determined enough to lead the way. This book is a good beginning.

MARTHA TEICHNER
CBS News Correspondent

Damascus, Syria
February, 1984

Introduction

How to Use This Book

This book is about a disability that affects not only the individual, but his family, friends, and the medical professionals to whom he turns for help. Most of the information in these pages will be useful to everyone affected by incontinence. But each of you may find special interest in those parts that deal with your particular problem.

If you are incontinent, you probably will want to begin with Chapter 2,"Personal Experiences." In it you will find that you are not alone. Others share your disability. There are strong social taboos about incontinence, but there are people who cope successfully. Strategies for coping, presented in Chapters 5 and 6, offer practical, forthright suggestions for adjusting emotionally, as does the chapter on sexuality (10). With this background, you should be able to begin your own management strategy. The medical and product chapters will provide you with ample references to plot a course of action.

If someone you love is incontinent, we suggest you begin your exploration of this book with Chapter 1, "Living with Problems of Bladder Control," and Chapter 3, "Attitudes Are the Real Disability." These chapters, followed by the chapter on personal experiences (2), will give you insight into the encompassing nature of incontinence. Prior to this point you probably have not completely understood what has been happening to your loved one, especially if family activities have been slowly and insidiously curtailed. Further understanding of what you have been experiencing can be achieved through reading the psychology sections.

If you are a professional—physician, nurse, social worker, nursing-home administrator, psychologist—please sit down and read the book straight through. The statistics tell us that you have clients, right now, who need the help offered within these pages. We challenge you to lead them to the help so many desperately need.

We at the Simon Foundation hope that this book and following editions will become dog-eared with use. And that the information you find within these covers will stimulate a process that will bring about change. Professional, family member, or incontinent person, each of us has a role to play in addressing this ignored disability.

Finally, we encourage you to act like children playing the age-old game of tag—pass it on.

1

Living With Problems of Bladder Control

Katherine Jeter, Ed.D., E.T.

One of my most vivid adult memories is our oldest child's third birthday. Early on that morning, twenty-two years ago, she began planning for the festivities later in the afternoon. As lunch time approached, Sally became more enthusiastic and more impatient. Soon frustration overtook anticipation and a temper tantrum ensued. As Sally stomped her little feet and wailed in exasperation at the delay, she forgot her recent training and wet her pants, and her socks, and the floor. She gasped in surprise and obvious embarrassment, and fled to her room. My maternal feet were planted in dismay and displeasure. How could she! How dare she!

Isn't it incredible that by the age of three a child is aware that involuntary loss of urine is unacceptable and cause for shame? Isn't it even more astonishing that a reasonably intelligent parent would be upset by a brief lapse in toilet training in a child so young? The fact is Western toilet rituals have long been passed from generation to generation and are stringently enforced. Trends in sexual behavior, breastfeeding, and women's roles may be as transient as musical fads; but our belief in the importance of the proper time and place for elimination is ingrained in our collective subconscious.

Many readers who select this book may be curious about the contributors. Beyond their medical, social-work, and psychology credentials, what has motivated them to focus on urinary incontinence? Not just to focus on it but to become fascinated with the problems associated with it and zealous in the quest for solutions to bring cure and comfort to those affected by it.

Early in my career as an enterostomal therapist in the Department of Urology at the Columbus-Presbyterian Medical Center in New York, I worked with many people who, for a number of reasons, were incontinent of urine. [Enterostomal therapy has now become a nursing specialty. ET nurses are trained to care for patients with ostomies, incontinence, draining wounds, and pressure sores.] Their stories still haunt me; their discomfort and inconvenience still energize me to look for improved methods of diagnosis and treatment, and for more successful ways to help the public understand the problem.

9

- Margaret told of having to change the route she walked from the subway to the building where she worked. The shortest way took her down a narrow windy street in midtown Manhattan. During the winter, when the cold wind whipped through her skirt and between her legs, the chafing from her incontinence pads was unbearable. From November until April, Margaret walked two extra blocks to avoid beginning her day in such misery.

- Tom's plight was just as serious, but his solution was hilarious. He had a large circle of friends who were not the least bit concerned about his bladder inadequacy. He was at the age when drinking beer was a status symbol and considered the mark of manliness. On Saturday nights, in the parks on the edge of the Hudson River in New Jersey, the chums would gather for camaraderie and booze. As the beer consumption increased, so did Tom's uncontrolled urinary flow. By nine o'clock Tom would have saturated all the pads he could wear and carry. His buddies, rather than curtail their fun, would help out in a pinch. They donated their undershirts for added absorbency.

- Sam's mother wanted him to lead a normal life, in spite of his incontinence. Hardly a day passed that she didn't create another ingenious solution to help her son manage his condition. One of her innovations merits recounting here. To enable Sam to have all the absorbent pads he would need for a whole day's outing at Yankee Stadium, she slit the lining seams of his raincoat. Inside the lining Sam's mother pinned dozens of pads. Since they were between the inner surface of the coat and the lining, no one could detect their presence. The whole idea sounds so good until one realizes how conspicuous the youngster would be wearing a raincoat on a warm sunny day in May.

In the early 1970s few incontinence products were available. Makeshift garments and devices often were more satisfactory than anything surgical suppliers had in stock. It seemed preposterous that we could be on the threshold of sending a man to the moon but could not devise a reliable means of collecting urine.

In fact, Dr. John K. Lattimer, then chairman of the Department of Urology at the Columbia-Presbyterian Medical Center, my boss and my mentor, suggested that we consult the National Aeronautics and Space Administration (NASA). Scientists there willingly shared their full report on waste management in space flight. During the Gemini program, despite the inordinate financial and engineering resources invested in the project, urine collection in the spacecraft was a persistent problem. We tried, on a much smaller scale, to emulate NASA's technique of making a custom mold of each patient's genital area to produce a latex garment that would fit exactly. Our lack of success was discouraging but not dissuading.

Next we turned to the leading manufacturers of urological instruments and medical devices—Dow, Johnson and Johnson, C.R. Bard, and others. They all asked the same questions: What is incontinence? Who is incontinent? How many are incontinent? And they all gave the same answer: There was no indication that enough people had the problem to justify the financial outlay required to conduct market research and begin product development.

That was ten years ago. Times have changed. Attitudes have changed, somewhat. Evidence of a more liberal society can be seen on bookstore shelves and television screens. Couples share the same bed in TV commercials and prime-time programs. Hemorrhoids and headaches are described and remedied. Toilet-bowl cleaners and antidiarrheals come into our den and living room as casually and frequently as Rolaids and Gravy Train.

In 1983, TV viewers saw advertised, for the first time, an absorbent garment for urinary incontinence. In 1985 Jameson Books, Inc., boldly released this book, admitting that selecting a title had been a worrisome challenge and that booksellers had not been universally enthused. Finally, after a decade of frustration, there is a forum for frank discussion of what might be termed "the last taboo." As this book makes its way to the shelves of popular bookstores, with an eye-catching dust jacket instead of a plain brown wrapper, the general public will realize that the problems of wetness, odor, and skin irritation associated with incontinence are shared by seven to twelve million Americans. An estimated 5 percent of the population suffer to some degree from bladder-control problems. An estimated 2 percent are affected seriously enough to require absorbent garments or devices. Once public awareness is heightened, the prevalence of the condition will be acknowledged. The pressure of sheer numbers will lead to new inquiry into the causes; improved medical and surgical solutions; more suitable products and devices; and, finally, elimination of the stigma that is responsible for this unspoken, unmentioned epidemic.

What is incontinence? Simply defined, it means passing body wastes in the wrong place involuntarily. Incontinence is not a disease. It is a symptom with many causes. Some health professionals refer to a person as being "slightly incontinent." That is like being "a little pregnant." The unexpected loss of urine in any amount, on a regular basis, in an inconvenient place is incontinence.

There are different types of incontinence. To determine the type and cause, a history will be taken to discover when and how much urine is lost. Urologists may want to do special diagnostic studies, called urodynamics.

The type of incontinence will dictate the appropriate treatment. Not everyone uses the same terminology. Among the problems of establishing definitions are individuals' perceptions. Two people may experience the same urine loss with the same frequency; one will consider it a slight nuisance, whereas the other will view it as a personal tragedy. The following framework was chosen for its simplicity:

Stress incontinence refers to leakage of small amounts of urine when coughing, sneezing, laughing, lifting, jogging, or doing anything that causes the abdominal pressure to override the bladder's closure mechanism. With all the talk about "stress" in the 1970s and '80s, it is important to emphasize that the physical stressors of stress incontinence should not be confused with the psychological stress of daily living.

Urge incontinence describes the compelling desire to urinate and the inability to delay voiding long enough to get to a toilet. Usually the embarrassed sufferer leaves a trail to the bathroom or a puddle on the floor. Sometimes the condition is especially aggravating because the urge to void occurs so soon after the bladder was emptied.

Overflow incontinence is the leakage of small amounts of urine without the urge to void or the inability to urinate normal volumes. As the term implies, the small amount of urine that exceeds the bladder's capacity runs off, but the bladder remains full. This condition can lead to damage in the urinary system.

Total incontinence is the complete absence of control, either continuous leakage or periodic uncontrolled expulsion of the bladder's contents. People who are mentally alert and physically able and who are contending with total urinary incontinence usually will beat down the doors of physicians until they find one who offers a medical or surgical cure for their problem.

Enuresis is the term most widely used to describe bedwetting in children who are old enough to be "potty-trained" and adults who have not gained control at night.

Incontinence may be the result of a birth defect, injury, disease, or the predictable anatomical and physical changes that occur with the aging process. Because it is a symptom, incontinence should be investigated to determine the cause . . . and the treatment.

Because intimate bodily functions have been such secretive, private subjects, it is not unusual to find that people have limited understanding of their urinary system. They may report they have "kidney trouble" when they mean to say they have "bladder trouble." A brief review will prepare our readers for the discussions to follow.

Most everyone is born with two kidneys. The kidneys filter impurities from the blood that flows through them with every heartbeat. The waste product they manufacture is called urine. Normally the kidneys produce about a quart of urine per day. The urine is transported down the ureters into the bladder, which is a muscular holding tank. In adults the bladder will hold eight to ten ounces before a signal that urination will soon be necessary is sent to the brain. Unless there is some abnormality, when the brain receives the message, it is able to consider several options. If a long road trip is scheduled to begin, a good choice would be to look for a toilet before starting out. If, on the other hand, one is in the midst of a romantic waltz on the dance floor, the urge can be suppressed until the music ends and it is comfortable to say, "Excuse me."

At the bladder outlet there is a muscle called a sphincter, which can be likened to a purse string. In its cinched position it prevents the passage of urine. Relaxed, it allows urine to pass through the urethra to the outside of the body.

The urinary system is normally sterile, that is, bacteria do not live in it. Normal urine does not have a foul odor. Its usual color is straw to pale yellow, but it varies according to the amount and type of food and drink consumed. Nothing more than these basic facts and this illustration is necessary to enjoy and profit from the chapters ahead.

Who is incontinent? Generally speaking, anyone who regularly has "accidents," day or night, past the age of three years, may be described as incontinent.

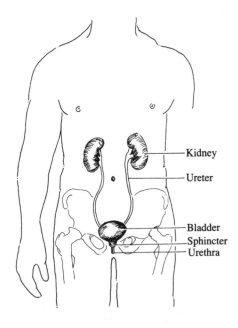

CHILDREN

Spina bifida (*spy*-na *bif*-i-da) is the most common crippling defect in children. The incidence of bladder and bowel incontinence with this condition is very high. There are other, lesser known conditions such as exstrophy of the bladder that interferes with urinary control and imperforate anus that may result in bowel incontinence.

An estimated one million children and adults are bedwetters. There are many theories about the cause of enuresis. Among the most popular is that enuretics sleep more deeply than other people and have a small-capacity bladder. Another popular contention is that the brain did not learn the proper signal during toilet training, or that it never got the signal in the first place.

The emotional toll that bedwetting takes is painful even to describe. Adults who have outgrown it remember youthful years of shame and withdrawal. Years when they could not attend or host slumber parties; when they couldn't go on overnight school outings; on camping expeditions into the vacant lot next door; or away to summer camp. They describe the various tactics their parents employed to "help" or "cure" them. Some were awakened every half hour all night for weeks and months. Some were made to swallow bitter potions every time they wet. Some had to do their laundry every morning and hang it outside on the line for all the neighbors to see. Others were made to sleep in the bathtub or on the bathroom floor so they would not soil the bedlinen. Perhaps the grimmest evidence of the importance we place on urinary control is the 1981 death of a South Carolina first-grader who, after wetting his pants, took more than the recommended amount of the medicine he had been given to help him achieve continence.

ADULTS

"In women past the age of forty," explains Dr. Roy Witherington of the Medical College of Georgia, "stress incontinence is a major health problem." Studies have shown that young women are also affected. Even those who have never borne children may regularly leak urine when they are giggling, running, and jumping. Many of these women wear sanitary napkins or wads of tissue in their panties and are too ashamed to complain to their doctor. It has been estimated that 8 percent to 25 percent of the sanitary napkins purchased are used for incontinence, not menstruation. Some investigators report that only one out of twelve persons who suffer from incontinence consults a physician.

Incontinence is a common malady among our growing elderly population. The causes are varied; and for many there are help and hope. Even when bladder control cannot be fully restored, comfort and security against leakage can be ensured. It is widely recognized that many older people are "put" into nursing homes simply because they are incontinent. It is a condition that may be disgusting to family members and even poorly tolerated by nursing personnel.

The percentage of males and females affected by incontinence shifts from age group to age group. More young males than females wet the bed. Incontinence is certainly more common among women in young adulthood and middle age. As men get older, and the prostate enlarges, urgency, frequency, and overflow incontinence are common symptoms that should not be ignored. When the prostate tissue that is narrowing the urethra is removed, urinary control is usually restored. Although most studies to date indicate that incontinence is more common among women than men over sixty-five, new data suggest that more men are affected than have been previously reported.

There are particular injuries and diseases that can be expected to result in impaired bladder function—either the inability to pass water or the inability to control the flow. Among them are spinal-cord injuries from war; automobile, diving, skiing, and motorcycle accidents; such things as multiple sclerosis; Parkinson's disease; diabetes; Alzheimer's disease; and stroke.

It is obvious, now, that incontinence can happen to anyone at any age. It is a symptom with many causes. How could such a common affliction have continued without acknowledgment for so long? Certainly the first and most logical reason is the "delicacy" of the subject. People have been too inhibited to discuss it.

In America we are still likely to be directed to the "powder room" or "men's room" instead of to the toilet. Slang terms such as "I need to make" and "I'm going to see a man about a dog" persist in certain geographical areas. These ridiculous euphemisms continue in the same communities and households where nudity and explicit sexual behavior appear uncensored on movie and television screens.

Apparently it is shame that stifles people's complaints about their condition. The public has remained unaware—and unconcerned—about the prevalence of urinary incontinence. When asked what he would do if his father came to visit and wet the bed on several occasions, the middle-aged son responded, "Oh, my dad would never do that." This was the same gentleman who wanted only cookie and beer commercials aired during sports programs because "problems that don't affect me shouldn't be forced on me via the TV."

Lack of public awareness results in low product sales which, in some cases, account for manufacturers' unwillingness to expand their product line. If customers aren't going to buy, producers are not going to produce.

The chasm between consumer and manufacturer is responsible, in part, for the delay in development of products people would welcome. The lack of communication may also be the root of some colossal misconceptions. Recently a researcher and a business consultant, both well informed on the subject of incontinence, expressed amazement that people were more interested in comfort and security than cost. One wonders what their priorities would be if *they* were to experience bladder leakage!

An array of products and packaging implies that the user is sick. The colors are hospital white and green. The design is unisex. It's as if the designers assume that loss of urinary control is accompanied by loss of personal pride and taste in wearing apparel.

Current third-party reimbursement (insurance) policies have not facilitated product development and distribution either. Many insurance companies do not reimburse for absorbent products. Inexplicably, the same insurance company that refuses to pay for absorbent pads may pay for an external collection device, such as a condom catheter. Medicaid pays for absorbent products up to a certain limit in some states but not in others. Some people are spending as much as a hundred dollars per month to keep dry and comfortable. On a fixed income, that is a large chunk of the budget.

What's to be done? Who's to do it? Two decades ago there was a similar "closet" condition called ostomy. People were having colostomies, ileostomies, and urostomies, but no one discussed them above a whisper. Many believed that they were synonymous with odor, flatulence, and baggy clothes to conceal a bulging appliance full of stool or urine. Now, such publicly known people as Al Geiberger, the professional golfer; Rolf Benirschke, the professional football player; and Tish Baldridge, the New York public relations consultant and former secretary to Jacqueline Kennedy Onassis, are assurances that an ostomy need not be an embarrassment or a limitation.

This change in attitude is the direct result of the tireless efforts of thousands of people with ostomies who, under the banner of the United Ostomy Association (UOA), have reached out to help prospective and newly operated patients. Dr. Ira Kodner of the Jewish Hospital in St. Louis has termed the UOA "the most successful consumer organization in health-care annals." An overstatement? Not when one considers that from its membership came the first enterostomal therapist and a nursing specialty called ET nursing. Not when one realizes the impact ostomy associations have had on product development and availability.

In some states the legislative activities of the ostomy associations have resulted in elimination of sales tax on ostomy appliances and accessories. In some areas of the country, it has been the ostomy associations that have both convinced hospitals to hire an ET nurse and provided the funds for the nurse's training.

It has been, in many instances, people with ostomies who have convinced surgeons of the importance of the location and dimensions of their abdominal stoma (the surgically created opening). Such lessons are not learned so easily from textbooks and professors.

Could such a groundswell of consumerism be replicated among people who are incontinent? Maybe. Maybe not. HIP, Inc. (Help for Incontinent People), was conceived with that intent in spring 1982. The first newsletter of helpful hints was published in winter 1983. When the HIP report was plugged in the "Dear Abby" column, thirty-five thousand people wrote for a subscription. And their letters continue at a rate of one hundred to two hundred per week. What are they saying?

- Until I read this article in "Dear Abby," I thought I was the only one with this kind of problem. Now it's like a load off my shoulders knowing that I don't have to feel so "alone" in this matter.

- I can't go to church anymore and that really hurts.

- . . . eighty-eight years old. For the past three years I have gone through "hell" being unable to hold my urine until I get to the bathroom. I have been confined to my home.

- I have spent a fortune in doctors and hospitals and still I don't have time to reach the bathroom when I have to go.

- I'm seventy-eight years old . . . get around good . . . but this trouble sure puts a crimp in my style.

- This is for my sixteen year old granddaughter with a problem. It's ruining her life.

- My urologist gave no help but left me with a feeling of disgust partly because of my overweight. My family doctor said he had the same problem—which didn't do me any good.

- I found doctors are not anxious to discuss the subject. I am tired of hearing, "Don't worry about it. We will get to that bridge when we come to it." Well, I crossed the bridge and I'm looking for news.

- When I mentioned it to my doctor he merely raised his eyebrows, said, "Oh," and promptly went on to another topic. So I must seek help elsewhere.

- Please send any helpful info . . . as I have to fly to Omaha to attend granddaughter's wedding. I'm ninety-one so would appreciate your help.

- I will be ninety in September. Do you think I am too old to try to get help as it has been a long time.

- I have endured three unsuccessful bladder operations so must spend many hard-earned dollars for sanitary pads. I am seventy years "young in heart."

17

- I don't have any serious bladder problem, but I'd like to have your newsletter so that I would be prepared in case I do have a problem.

- HELP! THANKS!

As eager as HIP members are to get and to share information, they still, for the most part, are reluctant to "come out." Efforts to hold meetings in several midwestern cities have been fruitless. Some people have listed their name as "Mr. Resident" or "Mrs. Occupant" to ensure that their confidentiality cannot be breached. Imagine what life would be like if we had been unwilling to acknowledge bad breath and body odor and look for remedies for these unsociable conditions!

It's 1984 now. We have an implantable artificial urinary sphincter. There are superabsorbent granules that can wick fifty times their own weight to increase security and capacity of incontinence garments. There are advertisements in newspapers and magazines. In recent months outlets such as K-Mart, Eckerd's, People's, Walgreen's have put large displays of incontinence products in a prominent position in their stores. Managers say that absorbent briefs, inserts, and underpads have begun "selling like hotcakes." There are continuing medical research and increasing interest among urologists, gynecologists, and geriatricians.

This is a brave new world and this a brave new book that will bring knowledge, comfort, and relief to thousands who have been disabled as much by the notion that theirs was a shameful condition as by the condition itself. As enlightened readers pass the news of new resources to friends and coworkers, self-help groups can't be far behind. And with them will surely come more innovative solutions for care and cure.

Personal Experiences—
People Managing Incontinence

Jill Balson, M.A.
Cheryle B. Gartley
John J. Humpal, Ph.D.

The people you will meet in this chapter might well be your neighbor, your teacher, your minister, or perhaps an aunt, mother, brother, or sister. Because these people who will be talking to you are like millions of other incontinent Americans, they are experiencing a disability that most people prefer to keep a secret. To keep their secret and avoid an embarrassing accident, they cope by curtailing their normal daily lives, often becoming totally isolated.

The following men and women, who range in age from fourteen to over seventy, have one thing in common: they are far enough along in their own adjustment to incontinence to be willing to talk about it. Oft times it wasn't easy. They cried, and we cried. Some expressed surprise at how difficult it suddenly became to talk when we clipped the microphone to the lapel. One person said he really didn't have much to say, and then talked for two hours straight.

From Arizona to Illinois, and Oregon to New Jersey, these are the people who let us into their lives. We will be forever in their debt.

TED . . . who ten years ago broke his neck in a freak accident. Today he has his own law practice.

SUE . . . who remembers vividly at age forty-five what it was like to be a bedwetter at age fourteen.

MARY JANE . . . a psychologist who has managed spina bifida and incontinence for forty years.

CHERYLE . . . who at the age of thirty began experiencing a series of severe urinary-tract infections whose sudden and unpredictable onset was accompanied by total incontinence.

MICHAEL . . . a sixth-grader who needed an artificial sphincter to remedy an incontinence problem caused by a birth defect.

NAN . . . Michael's mother.

JACK . . . an automobile accident victim who conquered his resulting disabilities and became a college professor.

DAYANN . . . a potential Miss America who at age sixteen has seen more of the bad side of human nature than most of us do in a lifetime. She uses clean intermittent catheterization to manage her incontinence.

STEVEN . . . a World War II disabled veteran. He finds his incontinence more difficult to manage than his confinement to a wheelchair.

JAMES . . . who took six months planning how to explain incontinence to his girlfriend, only to find out she thought it was no big deal.

SARAH . . . a grandmother and stroke victim who is able to joke with her grandchildren about having a grandmother who wears diapers and crawls.

VICKI . . . a peppy teenager, trying to hide incontinence protection under her skimpy cheerleading outfit, who lighted up our lives.

No matter their age, sex, the reason for their incontinence, or how well they were managing this disability, the people who joined in these conversations shared certain realities. They had to learn to deal with feelings of shame, loss of control, anger, exposure through intimate relationships, new medical procedures, fear, depression, the risk of accidents in public, and the ofttimes insensitive attitudes of others. Incontinence dominated their lives.

Mary Jane is a psychologist who has experienced incontinence all her life. She knows that what she recommends to her clients is not easy, nor is it without risk, but it is reality:

"Incontinence is a disability, just like any other, only there are more people who have it than people are aware of. The fact is, you can still go about a perfectly normal life. The bottom line of what I tell my patients when they are trying to deal with incontinence is that there are two ways you can deal with it.

"The first way, you can stay home and you won't have an accident in public. You can avoid dating and you won't be embarrassed around anybody that you care about. You can avoid doing all those things and nothing bad is going to happen to you and nobody is ever going to know . . . especially if you live alone . . . nobody's ever going to know. And you can spend your life like that. You know, I'll tell them all these negatives.

"Or, you can gamble. You can take a chance. You can take a chance that you'll get to know somebody and you'll go out with that person and maybe that person can't deal with your incontinence and you'll suddenly realize that you and that person aren't going to be able to make it. Just like when you went out with somebody before, and for whatever reason, that relationship didn't work. You can go to a job, and you can have an accident

20

and they can't put up with it. Maybe you'll lose that job because you feel self-conscious or maybe you'll find that you have better colleagues that you work with than you thought!"

When you first begin to manage your incontinence in order to return to a normal life, the task seems monumental. There wasn't a person among those who shared their stories who wasn't discouraged at first. But they fought their way back, each in his own way, to full productive lives. They felt that it is how we react to the circumstance of our lives that controls our destiny. That is what this book, particularly this chapter, is really about . . . choosing how our lives will be by choosing how we will behave.

THE OVERWHELMINGNESS

There is no denying that incontinence permeates all activities of one's life. Sometimes the feelings are so subtle one doesn't even realize they are there. Bringing these feelings from subconscious to conscious awareness is to begin the process of adjustment. Cheryle and Jill talk about just that.

> JILL: Then this all began three or four years ago for you, after you began having serious urinary-tract infections? When did it come to you that this was going to be something you were going to have to deal with?
>
> CHERYLE: I don't think it did. How's that for a dumb answer? I think what happened was that it was a sense of depression that set in before any logic set in. Not a gradual curtailing, not even realizing perhaps what you're doing. You just don't go out, anywhere. I just didn't live.
>
> JILL: What did you tell yourself? Why did you tell yourself you were doing that?
>
> CHERYLE: I don't think I did. That's what I'm really saying. I think the depression just took over . . .

Others, who didn't mention the depression, were always aware of their incontinence.

> JACK: Like, oh, it's hard to . . . it's hard to put into words unless you're going through it yourself. You know what I mean? For me to tell you what it's like. But the thing is that it's always there because you're aware of it.
>
> STEVEN: It takes time. It absorbs more than its allotted share of worry time, if you will. And it's a pain in the neck. A wheelchair really is not.

21

CHERYLE: I would not subject myself to having an accident in public. Even being out in the yard gardening was difficult. The neighbors would pounce on me—I think out of good intent—with questions about how I was feeling, and so on. Well, if you are right in the middle of a conversation like you and I are right now, you know, you just don't say—at least I couldn't—"You stand right here in this spot, I'll rush in and use the bathroom, and I'll come right back and I will remember exactly what point in the sentence you were at when you were telling me how your mom's dying of cancer." Those are the kinds of burdens incontinence brings. What do you say to somebody?

So what you come up with is incredible, total isolation—self-imposed and desired—rather than face the problem. But not thought through as to what you are doing to your life. In some ways, I hear you repeatedly trying to get me to tell you what decisions I made. At the level that I understand decisionmaking, I made none. I just acted.

You get into somebody's car, and you are relieved to see that they have leather or vinyl seats. I mean, the stupidity of it all. Or you won't get into somebody's car because you know it's a brand new car and you're not going anywhere in that.

If I'm going out—if I'm *willing* to go out, that is—bike riding or something, you always have two blouses on. You know, a T-shirt-type thing with a blouse, which would look very natural tied around your waist if you had an accident, right? How many bikers, joggers, etc., do you see dressed that way, with something around their waist. In dress clothing you're stuck. Who's going to take his business jacket off and tie it around his waist? The thought has crossed my mind! I guess in terms of living, I would say that incontinence *governs your whole life*.

MARY JANE: I was always fearful of trying something or doing something new because I was afraid of having an accident. I would not go to somebody's house as a child and stay all night. Everybody came to my house to stay with me. I would not go someplace else and wet on somebody else's bed.

I choose to work where I do now because it's so close to where I live that I can go home and change clothes. It does dictate my whole life.

In college I washed clothes in the middle of the night, two or three o'clock in the morning, I did that—because I didn't want to carry wet stinky laundry down to the laundry room when everybody was down there washing clothes. I washed almost every other day because you couldn't let towels build up in your room or you had a smell problem.

22

After all, you had a roommate to deal with. You didn't want to put her out with this thing.

So I was considered very weird down there washing clothes, waiting until the dorm was empty at four o'clock in the morning to go down to the laundry room.

These people sound pretty overwhelmed, don't they? They probably were. But if you look again closely at what they are saying you will see the tiny beginnings of coping with incontinence. Beginnings that turned these people into psychologists, teachers, businessmen, lawyers, people living again.

THE ANGER

Elizabeth Kübler-Ross, in her book about death and dying, speaks about anger as a legitimate emotion. It is also a legitimate and healthy emotion when coping with incontinence. Whether it is chronic or temporary, incontinence represents a personal loss. Anger allows you to recognize that loss and grieve for it. Through allowing the anger to come out, you also learn to recognize what it can't do for you. To remain stuck in a state of anger means for most people to remain without other coping mechanisms that might help to dissolve the feelings of futility and hopelessness.

Mary Jane, who has lived with incontinence all her life, says: "So I always thought it was me that God picked out for this wonderful thing. And until I got around, got older and saw people who had disabilities that involved incontinence, it came as a big shock to me that it wasn't the most unusual thing in the world. Then I became a little angry at teachers and people who hadn't known anything about it. They made me feel so unusual."

It doesn't matter if you lived with incontinence all your life, or if it's a new challenge. People still get angry when it happens to them.

"I've almost gotten to the point," says Cheryle, "where I get so angry that I want to carry this paraphernalia and be blatant about it. You know, go get T-shirts made that say I leak, I'm incontinent, or whatever. You just get so mad you want to say to yourself, OK, I'll drive myself to bust through this mindset. Yet I know I won't. I could go through all that craziness and it wouldn't change the mindset in any way. It might get me a little publicity, which I didn't want. It wouldn't get you anything else."

Other people who care about the person who is incontinent get angry too. Cheryle had this to say about a friend who got angry about incontinence: "And I think that his anger helped. I can remember him saying to me, some comment about how he just didn't understand, that there must be other people with this problem. It was both a general anger and kind of an anger

23

at me which said, 'C'mon, kid, you're a bright girl. What the hell are you doing? Why isn't this problem fixed . . . why do you want me to believe that man can walk on the moon and you have to stay in your home?' "

Sometimes people sound as if they are just giving up, when in fact they are really angry. Jack sounds like a quitter, but he managed to get an advanced degree and become a professional: "I don't get out that much anymore, you see. And sometimes, honest to God, I just get tired. I just get tired—I'm tired of fighting. Because it seems like the whole thing has been a fight just to survive with some kind of dignity. And you get tired of fighting; you get tired of these attitudes.

"But like I said to you, that stuff, the anger, the bitterness, it's just all a waste of time. It's a waste of energy you need to save in order to cope."

Greater perhaps than the feelings of anger, pervasiveness, isolation, and depression are the fear and the associated feelings about the possibility of having an accident in public.

FEAR AND SHAME

SUE: What I remember, of course, is the shame. The one accident I do remember was in first grade. The teacher was very intolerant of this kind of thing. Nobody belongs in school if they don't have this under control, and it was a matter of, you know, pointing the finger and her saying "bad girl" and intentionally humiliating me in front of the others.

MARY JANE: The first time I had an accident at college, I wasn't going to go back the next day. I had already paid my tuition but that didn't matter. My folks said I needed to try to return. I really wasn't going to go back the next day, I was just too humiliated. Well, I went back and it wasn't that big a deal.

VICKI: When I was fifteen, I became a cheerleader and discovered a problem which was very frustrating. At times when I would jump or kick I'd have a sudden panicked feeling that I was nearly wetting my pants. Running in and out of the gym is not a good image for a cheerleader so I would wear the heaviest feminine pads I could find. This was anything but pleasant, especially wearing such bulk under a slight cheerleading uniform. It gave me a little more assurance, though. The mere thought of wetting while cheering in front of a crowd filled me with terror.

CHERYLE: One accident is enough to scare you to death. After an accident, I remember one job I had which demanded that I be out from the workplace for four or five hours every day entertaining customers; it was part of the job. And I would come home from work with a headache every day because I had so severely dehydrated myself in order to avoid an accident. Absolutely guaranteed that by four o'clock in the afternoon I had a blinding headache.

JAMES: When you have an accident you wish you could just go poof and disappear.

JACK: I remember the worst accident I have had. My attendant did everything right except he didn't hook the catheter to the leg bag. You know what I mean? I'm sitting in class and suddenly I hear running water, and there was a puddle underneath my desk, you know, it was like running from the catheter. That was probably the most embarrassing moment, because there were so many people who were probably looking around and thinking hey, there's water running somewhere.

Like I say, if you're ready to go out and something happens, you're not going to be in a very good mood, especially if an accident ruins your time out. I don't get out that much to begin with.

DAYANN: The teacher was mad at us and said nobody is allowed to leave this classroom even to go to the bathroom. And this one boy, his name was _____, and he just blurted out my problem and the whole class was silent. And the principal was right there. It really killed me. The principal didn't do anything. [Crying uncontrollably again.] Neither did the teacher. He said, "Well, Dayann has . . . Dayann wets her pants, so you have to let her go." That really killed me because it was blurted out in front of the whole class. And the adults didn't do anything. I'm about in tears and everything, and they did nothing.

Because of what happened last year, I'm afraid it might replay itself.

CHERYLE: That's a good phrase, by the way. Replay itself. That's what it would seem like, wouldn't it? Like a nightmare come back.

DAYANN: No, it would be a nightmare come true!

FEAR OF ACCIDENTS

Accidents are part of living with incontinence, and the fear of having one, as you can see by the above statements, is a very normal reaction to managing incontinence.

JILL: I've never heard anybody say—and I don't expect to hear anybody say—oh, well, it doesn't matter, I'll have an accident.

CHERYLE: You're never going to hear that out of me.

JILL: I am never going to hear it out of anybody. It does matter.

CHERYLE: Yes, it certainly does matter. Perhaps when this problem has been discussed openly for several years, then people will find less horror in it. They might find more ability to avoid having it govern their lives 100 percent of the time if we talk about it and accept it as a society, if we learn to talk about it in the family room, and if we learn to bring some acceptance to it. I think that the people who suffer from it, instead of their life being governed by incontinence 100 percent of the time, maybe the problem will only govern 10 percent of their life.

JILL: Do you really believe that?

CHERYLE: Yes. But I don't believe there'll be a person who will ever say in my lifetime that it doesn't matter if I have an accident. I don't think that's within the human capability. Not in the way that we are all developing; it is just not possible.

CONTROL

Lack of control was a major theme running through all of our conversations. Being incontinent causes people to feel their life is very much out of control. Returning to feeling some sense of being under control was a priority for many. Control is a legitimate human need that can be dangerously counterproductive if it is poorly expressed.

JACK: Incontinence makes you aware of how little control you have. We're in this world where there's little enough control as it is over our lives. I mean what with nuclear weapons and all the other stuff. And then, when you can't even do that, you really feel helpless.

MARY JANE: Well at the time I went through these experimental surgeries on my bladder, I was fourteen. I was in the teenage years and wanted to be like other kids. The main problem stopping me from socializing and being very self-conscious was bladder problems. I probably would have hung from a tree by my toes if they told me it would bring me control.

CHERYLE: Incontinence governs every yes or no response to invitations; it governs all of them. Well, it's really the control mechanism, you know. In fact, psychologically, I have no idea what my personality would be like without having dealt with this disability. Control is one of the things that I've often disliked in myself, and now I see other people do it when they are in the same life circumstances. You are always looking for control. I'll drive. I'll meet you there. Let's have the meeting at my house. Let me set the time. I look at other personalities who are so flexible and I think, I must look like the world's worst bitch.

MARY JANE: That's one of the things that I learned to do. I volunteered so that I had control and everything was at my house. So I found that I could control the environment and that I wasn't afraid if I was controlling the situation.

Franklin D. Roosevelt's observation that "there is nothing to fear but fear itself" is relevant to incontinence. Those who fear having an accident in public do have an option since there is a way to dissipate the fear. Webster defines an accident as an unforeseen or unplanned occurrence, and unexpected happening. Given this definition of accident, we who are incontinent should never have an accident again, because we can foresee the event, we can plan for it, we can expect what will happen, and we can be prepared to cope with the unexpected loss of urine.

SURVIVAL

There is no one right way to cope with being incontinent, or with the public attitudes on incontinence. Some people try to understand social attitudes: some find humor even in the most stressful situations; others join support groups. The challenge is to find whatever works for you and is constructive, so that you can get on with living. Others shared with us how they coped and didn't cope with incontinence.

JILL: You had to give people excuses. What was your excuse for not going anywhere?

CHERYLE: Busy. I'd say no thank you, I'm busy. In fact, you are one of the few people that I really gave an honest answer to when you extended a dinner invitation. And your response was, well if you are having incontinence problems that night, we will come to your house. And I can remember saying to you, what, and watch me change clothes all evening?

MARY JANE: Kids associate going to the bathroom with intelligence. If you're too dumb to go to the bathroom, you're pretty stupid. So you tend then to become a show off in other ways. That's how I coped when I was little. I found myself deliberately learning some subjects in school that kids who were particularly obnoxious to me were good at. I would go out of my way to go to the library and learn everything about something they thought they knew so much about just to put them down. Because they had been implying that because I was incontinent, I was stupid.

JILL: That's a good coping mechanism, isn't it? I mean, it got you somewhere.

MARY JANE: Violence. Right up there with violence! At school, they were walking around in nylon dresses with ruffles and petticoats all the time. My mother had to be able to wash my clothes, with bladder accidents she just washed and washed and washed clothes. I had dresses that would only be worn one time because I wanted something I'd see in a store. You know you can't have an accident in a felt skirt with a poodle on it and wear it again!

When I was a teenager I used to cope by telling a lot of lies. If somebody would invite me to something that I was kind of scared to go to, a late party at somebody's house where people might stay over, I would tell them I had a date with this person that nobody else knew and make up all kinds of stories about him. So that they didn't think that I was just going to stay home by myself.

Now I think I cope much more constructively. I tend to tell people a lot about me before I start going out with them. That way there are no surprises or awkwardness.

Coping with incontinence is not only adjusting your own psychology to the disability, not only planning for accidents in public, but also taking charge of having a positive self-image, being self-confident and being responsible for one's own self-esteem. "It's not easy," Linda says, "I think it's just getting out into the world and making people aware that you're there and you have just as much right to live as anybody else does, you know?"

SEXUALITY

Continuing to function as a sexual being is also a very important part of taking steps to have a positive self-image. Incontinence is not sexuality, no matter how often the two are confused.

JAMES: I'm incontinent, not impotent. The only thing the two have in common is they both begin with the letter *i*.

MARY JANE: A lot of people confuse incontinence with the sexual— you can have one problem and not the other. They may write you off sexually because you can't use your bladder, like a girlfriend of mine who assumed I didn't have a period. I use to look at people like that as, boy, are you stupid! Until I realized that they don't really understand incontinence.

Mary Jane, ever the realist, has good advice when it comes to incontinence and sexuality: "I wouldn't mind so much being married; I find the idea of sexuality and all really kind of exciting and interesting. However, the thought of waking up with somebody in a wet bed does cross your mind, like how long is this guy going to like you? At first it seemed like it would sort of take some of the luster off of the wedding. I found when I starting counseling people, this is a big issue. What is he or she going to do when he or she finds out about these problems.

"I tell them to change the sheets. The quality of a marriage or relationship doesn't get based on an accident or something that happens from time to time. What destroys a relationship is lack of communication. They don't talk about what they are feeling, they don't talk about the issues, they don't even talk about how they feel about the accident. Sometimes people don't even do things that keep romance alive."

JACK: I've had to really be honest with myself about women and sexuality. I said, hey, after fifteen years, what is it? I mean, you got a lot of friends, and they tell you you're a nice guy, you have a nice personality, and you're not extremely ugly. What is the problem? So maybe it's not me. I'll put the problem on the back of the women of America, because maybe it's their problem. If you watch any TV at all or read the papers, people are bombarded; they are told what to want, what is desirable, and this and that. And if a person is prey to that kind of outside influence, well obviously, I'm not the kind of man every mother would want her daughter to go out with. Right?

CHERYLE: I've often thought that if there was anyone who could handle it well enough to suit me, to make me comfortable—you know, first of all that's discounting whether it's the other person's job to make you comfortable or not. I can't help but wonder if there is anyone who could react in such a way that would make it all comfortable. I don't have an answer to that except to know that it really isn't their responsibility to react in a certain way.

NAN [on sex education for her child]: And I guess at this point I don't want for Michael to start seeing himself as being different sexually. Now, I have some questions myself and I don't want to give him any false information. I know he can have an erection, but will he leak urine? So what we've talked about has been just a normal kind of sex education. I guess I just don't know where to get the information I need.

SARAH [in a letter]: I absolutely cannot imagine being sexually involved—in this matter incontinence is a real handicap. [This from a woman who continues:] Yes, all of the family knows about the problem and sometimes they and my friends who know of it remind me that perhaps I had better take a few minutes to check things out. Once in

29

a while I will joke with one of my grandchildren about having a grandmother who wears diapers.

As the above glimpses show, there is no doubt that attitudes about sexuality and incontinence are complicated and often difficult to deal with. James and Dayann deserve the final statements on sexuality because they are so healthy.

James spent *six months* figuring out just exactly how to break the news to his first special girlfriend, only to find out she barely had six minutes of curiosity over the topic. James remarks: "So that helped me build up confidence. She accepted *me*. Women are going to have to deal with it if they really want me. I am what I am. That's it. It won't go away."

Dayann says: "My counselor told me when I get a boyfriend that I really can trust, then I can tell him all about my problem and stuff. And if he can't understand it, then he's not the right one for me. I think she's right. Because if he can't accept that, then he can't accept me, you know?"

ATTITUDES

Attitudes about sexuality and incontinence have a wide range from a matter-of-fact "change the sheets" to "no, absolutely not." In fact, no matter what the topic we discussed with people who were incontinent, attitude was the pivot point on which all actions and behavior turned. All of us live out our own values and those of the society that has shaped us.

It would benefit all of us, those who are incontinent today, and those who may face it later, to work toward improving our cultural norms and attitudes about this topic. Jill and Nan talk about this very thing:

> JILL: How did you tell him that incontinence was all right, that he was okay but we're still not going to tell anybody about this. We are going to keep it a secret?
>
> NAN: We talked about the fact that people are foolish and dumb, ignorant. That other children are not going to understand this. That most people are ignorant, and that they think a person wearing a Pamper is a baby.
>
> JILL: Laid it at the door of other people?
>
> NAN: Yes, which in fact is where the responsibility lies. And if society were more enlightened, we wouldn't have to have a family secret like this. But society is not enlightened, and we do not intend for Michael to be the one in school to do it. Because we know it will be traumatic. So he's just known that most people just don't understand having an artificial sphincter.

I have a friend who suggested that maybe—maybe kids would be more understanding than we think. And she may be right. I don't know. I guess I just don't want to take the chance, because then again she may be wrong. And I've only got one chance. You know, I'm just interested in the adjustment of one little boy named Michael.

JACK: You have to be tough. You have to make yourself tough or you die. You may not die physically, but you die inside; your spirits become so broken that you just become a shrinking violet where every little thing would just send you up a wall.

It's amazing what goes on in people's minds. Sometimes I sit here, away from the world, and think about how little character there is left in the world today. Because just so many people are mean-spirited.

ADVICE

Despite some of the insensitive attitudes people feel from society around them, the people we have been talking to have learned to live with incontinence, to return to a normal daily life—school, work, church, social functions. For most of us, isolation is no way to live, yet at one time or another, all of these people used reclusiveness and isolation to adjust to incontinence. We asked them for advice to help others.

CHERYLE: First and foremost, depression won't help you to adjust. Never helped anybody do anything. If you recognize that you're depressed, get help for it. I would guess that depression is probably the number one disability in this country. For many people it is correlated with incontinence because incontinence changes your life. And of course depression keeps you from functioning in terms of using your intellect to solve your problem.

Second, and this is *very important*, I think that one cannot get reality from people if you do not put reality out there. Meaning, had I said no thank you to you too many times when you invited me to dinner, together we would have distorted reality. I would have been giving you misinformation, and you would have over time, I think, felt rejected enough that no friendship would have ever developed. But when I gave you reality, I got reality back. I didn't reject you, and, lo and behold, you didn't reject me. So unless one is willing to put life into reality terms, I don't think one will ever go forward in their adjustment to incontinence. It's not that I am unaware that from time to time you will get some bad input from people using this approach. But life is full of risk. It isn't just dealing with incontinence that makes life risky.

Third, try to solve the problem. Look for a physician who takes kindly to it and look at every possible solution you can. Don't accept what doesn't need to be accepted. You know that old prayer, "God give me the strength to know the difference."

TED: But the best advice you can say is you just have to go on with the rest of your life. This is going to be a major headache for as long as you live. Just deal with it day to day and go about your life. You can't allow this to run you. There are still plenty of things you can do, places to go, people to see. You can work, you can make your way in the world as long as you don't let those problems overcome you.

I think that's really important. You just got to look at incontinence as a nuisance, you know. And try to keep perspective, and say to yourself that everybody's got their problems in one way or another.

DAYANN: You have to be careful of what you think of yourself. Think of yourself as just normal, just like other people. You are the same person you were before you had this problem. I don't think of myself as underprivileged or anything. I just think of myself as another human being. That's how I'd tell grownups who get incontinence to behave. It works for me.

When you can take Dayann's advice and again think of yourself as just like other people, a realization will dawn on you. "Normal" people tend to have so much to deal with in their own lives that they are not really focused on your incontinence—it's *you* that focuses on incontinence.

Mary Jane tells us about this in relating a tale about one of the groups she runs for people who are adjusting to life in a wheelchair:

"The one person who sticks out in my mind of all the groups I have run was a guy who really wanted to go to Chicagofest. When the rest of the group asked him how he liked the concert he admitted he hadn't gone because he didn't want everyone staring at him being there in a wheelchair. I pointed out that I was there and there were at least fifteen or twenty people in wheelchairs.

"He replied, 'I went every year before my accident and I've never seen any.'

"I said, 'If you've never seen any wheelchairs, it's because you weren't into wheelchairs last year.' And it hits them. It's the very same with incontinence. People who have just begun dealing with incontinence, weren't into it last year.

"As you get older, just plain age in life or experience, you suddenly realize people are so into themselves it doesn't occur to them what your little crisis is over there in the corner."

32

Sidney J. Harris, the columnist, summarizes Mary Jane's concept quite well in one of his columns: "Most of what is popularly called an 'inferiority complex' is really a form of vanity: the vanity of thinking that people are thinking about you, when they are busy thinking about themselves."

3

Attitudes Are the Real Disability
Cheryle B. Gartley

Jory Graham, who in her lifetime did a great deal to change the attitudes toward those living with the chronic disease called cancer, once said, "I can do nothing about the basic problem. The fact is that scientists do not yet know what causes cancer and therefore do not know how to guarantee its cure. But I can affect the social climate. I can fix responsibility. I can help bring about sanity and compassion and fair play."

For many, incontinence is a chronic disability, not unlike living with cancer. Incontinence too deserves an enlightened social climate. Sanity, compassion, and fair play are experiences that help many people overcome the barriers of their handicap. Unfortunately for all of us, society has not yet learned to cope with incontinence in this manner. In fact, human kindness often vanishes when confronted with urinary malfunction. Not the least among those whose unconscious cruelty lacerates the incontinent are the doctors and nurses to whom they turn for help.

A WORD ABOUT AND TO THE MEDICAL PROFESSION

People who are incontinent are living with a difficult, chronic problem. Some of them have been searching for help for many years, others have agonized for months getting up the courage to seek help. When they arrive at a doctor's office, clinic, or hospital, they carry with them a hope, a hope for compassion, understanding, and a solution. Do they leave with their self-image intact, with renewed energy to address this problem, with hope for a solution? Most of the people with whom we spoke in Chapter 2 had something to say on this topic.

> JACK: The urologists that I've been involved with were basically concerned with my ability to empty my bladder. Okay. But that's only part of the problem. But as far as skin care or continence, it just didn't seem to have been a concern of theirs. I guess it seemed to them if you want to take care of it, just put an internal catheter in.
>
> If all you need is someone to help you put your pants on, that's one

thing. But when it gets down to sanitation, you're talking about the basics in life. You're going back to birth, man; that's what you do with babies. And so once the hospital staff starts seeing you as a dependent baby, they start treating you as one. Where people require this kind of care, the staff begins talking to them like the village idiot: "You have to go to the washroom now, dear . . ."

NAN: I wish that I could challenge a roomful of doctors to take a week off and follow their patients. Start at home in the morning. Come, go to school with Michael for a day. Pick another child, pick a mother with a two-year-old in a spica cast that's been soaked with urine and smells, and follow her through her day. Find out what their life is like. Obviously they don't do that. They see you in the office for maybe three minutes. You throw yourself in front of the door so they can't get away. And they don't see your child at his desk when he's normal, when he's not crying because he's scared. They don't know what you live with. I don't think they'd be so cavalier in some of their suggestions if they took time to do this. But they don't.

Doctors are so into the whole medical scientific thing that many have completely disassociated that from emotional mental well-being on the part of the patient. Little things. Like they don't talk to Michael, they talk to me. He's twelve years old; don't ask me how he's doing, ask him.

When he was a little baby, one time, some resident said to me, "Oh, what a cute smile." Well, I just floated home the rest of the day, and I thought after that, there's always something good to say about a child. Even if the doctor just said what beautiful brown eyes your child has, it's something. Give me something positive when you're dumping all this negative on me. I think medical schools ought to have a class taught by someone like Cheryle, or the mothers of handicapped kids who could and would say some of these things to doctors.

INTERVIEWER: As a society we have put the medical profession on a pedestal. I think sometimes that we only do that because they have our lives in their hands. So we want to think that they are more special. Wouldn't we feel terribly insecure if we really knew, as my husband always says, half of them graduated at the bottom half of their class.

NAN: Yes we do that. We want them to know all the answers, and I think we put ourselves in an inferior position. We say, you are superior, you have an M.D.; I am a lowly person, I'm not that well educated; therefore, you must be right. But part of me in my innermost being is saying no. That's not right for me. I've seen this in my family and I know what our needs are.

I find among pediatricians and family doctors a more humble kind of attitude than among specialists. The more into this you get, specialists, neurosurgeons, and all, they always have the little entourage behind them. They *never* come in alone. They always come in with a couple of residents. You never know who they are. You know, five or six sort of come into the room together, and there's this awesome presence, and they have to perform for their entourage.

LINDA: I don't know if it's possible, but I think the whole medical outlook should be a little bit different. I think that they should maybe listen to the patient a little bit more. If they would listen, maybe they could heal.

Healing is such a wonderful word that there seems to be accomplishment built right into the sounds of it. I hear other words when someone says healing, words like trust, empathy, and a joint effort. The joint effort of the patient and the doctor looking for a solution, managing a problem, but not necessarily finding a cure. The difference is very important, especially when one is talking about a potentially chronic disability such as incontinence.

The thought processes are molded and shaped when a person pursues a medical degree. Ofttimes physicians expect that they will totally solve the patient's problems or that it is beyond the human capacity to fix, such as terminal diseases. Incontinence, like other chronic disabilities, often falls through the cracks, because the patient stays symptomatic and returns. In the case of incontinence, healing may mean management. A new way of thinking about such chronic problems should be developed by the whole profession.

A very able nurse who works with a renowned neurosurgeon stated the need for this chapter in no uncertain terms. She felt strongly that physicians, like all people on the job, need feedback. However, most feedback they receive is positive; the nurses and staff get the complaints.

A NATIONAL ATTITUDE

The phrase "attitudes are the real disability" is the theme of a lecture given by one of the authors of this book, Henry Holden. The phrase has become extremely meaningful to those of us working with the emotions and attitudes surrounding the topic of incontinence. We've explored the behavior of the continent part of the human race through the eyes of the incontinent. Their stories and experiences shed light on a national attitude that is unhealthful to us all.

One mother of a child with a physical disability makes a point of visiting the new teacher every fall to explain her son's condition and urge the teacher to have normal expectations of the child. The mother does not mention the child's associated incontinence partly because of the reactions like the following:

"His third-grade teacher was a real jerk. I knew that from the beginning from my little encounter before school started in the fall. She told me how nervous she was about having my son in her classroom, and I thought, this'll be a real good year. She was to call me if she needed any help or had any questions, but she never did. At the end of the year I saw her in the hall and she stopped me and said: 'This hasn't been too bad a year after all. I think I could even have one of those kids in a wheelchair in my class, but between you and me, it's those kids that can't go to the bathroom that I couldn't handle.'

"I just turned away and smiled. I thought, lady, you are a real fruitcake, and I'm so glad my son is out of your class. He's had a diaper all year, you dumb, dumb woman."

The frustrations of trying to help a loved one deal with incontinence are normal and to be expected. People who cope well 90 percent of the time do fall apart and make mistakes. Dayann talks about an incident she remembers clearly:

"When I have an accident at school I don't want to come home and change because then my parents would know. They think I'm too old for that stuff. They understand that I have a problem, but they just want me to train myself better so it will go away. What they don't seem to understand is that I'm going to have this problem for the rest of my life. Last year my dad made me write a thousand times, 'I will not wet my pants.' He doesn't do that anymore, but I remember. I guess he thought it was the only way to get me to stop. And it never does."

The understanding Dayann didn't find at home was found in a friend whose attitudes have made all the difference: "She understands it. I think that she is the only one, because she can tell me honestly how she feels about it. She can say it in such a nice way. It doesn't really seem to bother her, because she is different. She's not really strange or anything, just different."

"How do you mean different?" I asked.

"Well, she's nice to everybody. I mean really nice. She can't stand being mean to anyone."

"You're right, that is different!"

Sometimes incontinence is a result of other disease processes such as cancer or a stroke. People who are incontinent because of this often need help with personal care. Jack talks about two different helpers he's experienced, their different approaches to the problem, and what this meant to him:

37

"There was this one attendant that I had. He was very understanding. He would drop what he was doing to come up to my room at college and help me. I'd be apologizing all over the place and he would say, 'Hey, it's my job.' And he made it less embarrassing.

"But I've had just the opposite reactions. My own sister does it to me all the time; when she changes my bag she starts gagging. I think to myself, thanks a lot. She says she can't help it and maybe she can't."

When friends, relatives, and associates are understanding and helpful, what a difference it made.

> JANET: We went to a party at his friend's house one time and the catheter came off. His friends were real good about it too. They didn't make him feel like a fool or like that's really disgusting or anything like that. They took it really well. We really felt we could do things with this group of people again.
>
> STEVE: I have a couple of friends with cars: they will take me home to change if I have an accident; they even cooperate in saying that we are going after cigarettes, so no one will know what really happened. They are really good friends.

Mary Jane had an accident at work and immediately went home. She was determined that she wasn't going back. "They called me from work, one of the secretaries did, and said that she and another coworker had cleaned up the chair. The chair's fine. We just scrubbed it down, you know; it's no big deal. So I went back to work; nobody seemed the least bit different. In fact, they gave me reports that I hadn't finished typing the day that I left. Nobody made that big a deal out of it."

Mary Jane also remembers very favorably a boyfriend who experienced several accidents with her: "We were very close for a long time because of experiences that made for such good stories. His attitude was, well, okay, there was incontinence, but it was just part of our time together; you know, like one of the bad things that happens with the good things in life. When other people came along, often they didn't meet my standard of David. You know, I realized that I didn't have to feel sorry for myself or go out with losers because I had this trouble with incontinence and it was all I could get."

David made life fun for everyone around him. Once he purchased tickets to a play for them and was unable to get aisle seats. When Mary Jane was unable to leave her seat during the performance she had an accident. David, ever the quick thinker, had an accident himself. He poured his orange pop into her lap, then sat back and enjoyed himself while everyone around them helped her clean up and talked about what a clumsy date this adorable girl had.

Fun aside, many of the people who were both incontinent and in a wheelchair stated that the inability to walk was less of a problem than their incontinence. This didn't surprise Nan at all: "Because I think of the image . . . a wheelchair is socially acceptable. And becoming more so. I mean there are wheelchair athletes who race in marathons, and they are visible. They are written up in the *New York Times*. There are many of these programs, and people seem to feel, hey, isn't he neat. Even the abled-bodied world respects these people. There is nowhere in our society that it's acceptable or where you are given respect for being incontinent."

Managing incontinence, like regaining the use of a limb after a stroke, is a challenge. Fortitude, courage, and never-ending determination are required. Victory over this disability deserves the same respect—no more, no less—as all other life challenges met and conquered. Attitudes *are* the real disability.

Dayann says, "Well, if you have an accident in public, people think you have a mental handicap instead of a physical handicap. So they'll be real nice to you and talk real slow. I've had people come up to me and ask, what's wrong with you? Often this will happen when I am out shopping, so I tell them about my injury and they say, 'Oh, I'm so sorry,' I've heard that from a thousand people, 'Oh, that's so terrible; I do hope you get better,' I say—"

"Say, why thank you. I hope you get better too!"

"I never say that," replied Dayann, laughing, "Maybe someday I'll try it. After all, how else are people going to get changed if no one helps them, and I *do* hope they get better!"

Leo Buscaglia in his introduction to *Personhood* says it best: "Like the spider, there are those of us who refuse to stop spinning, even when it would appear to be far more sophisticated to be without hope. Our rope, though perhaps frail, can still be spun with optimism, curiosity, wonder, love, and the sincere desire to share a trip to the stars. Our goal is worth the struggle, for in this case the star to which we aspire is full humanity for all. I feel strongly that in the continual striving for actualization of every living thing lies our only hope."

4

How Your Urinary System Functions

Jean Cavanaugh, M.D.

The purpose of this chapter is to help you understand what is happening to your body. This in turn will help you discuss your case with your physician and other medical personnel. With education and understanding, you, the patient, can become your own strongest ally, and can prevent complications instead of being treated after the fact.

NORMAL ANATOMY AND PHYSIOLOGY

To begin with, let's get a good picture of what is happening during normal bladder emptying, or micturition, as the medical profession calls it. Figure 1 shows where the kidneys and bladder are in relation to the outside of your body. The kidneys are nestled snugly up against your back just below the rib cage. (This is why you get back pain if you have a bladder infection

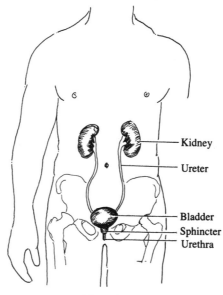

Figure 1

that grows into a more severe kidney infection. If you begin to have such pain, you should definitely call your physician.) The ureters are tubes that connect the kidneys to the bladder, which is situated in the lowermost part of the abdomen or pelvis. Normally you cannot feel the bladder, but if it is full of urine you may feel a fullness in the midline above the pelvic bones. The urethra empties the urine from the bladder. In males the urethra passes through the prostate, which can cause obstruction and inadequate emptying of the bladder.

Urine is formed in the kidneys and emptied through the ureters into the bladder. Please refer to figure 2 to help follow the pathways I will be

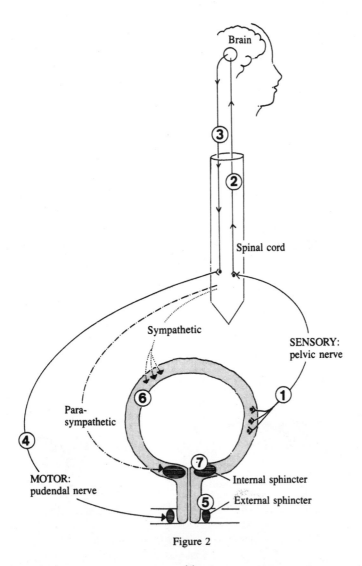

Figure 2

describing. The diagram has been simplified to depict the way the system works rather than the true anatomy itself. The bladder fills slowly and distends, or enlarges. When the bladder muscle is distended enough, sensory nerves detect this; then sensory nerve fibers via the pelvic nerve (1) transmit this urge to void to the spinal cord, where other nerves (2) transmit this message to the brain. The brain then sends a message back down the spinal cord (3) and out through a peripheral nerve, the pudendal nerve (4), to the external sphincter (5). The external sphincter is a skeletal or voluntary muscle like any other muscle in our arms or legs which we think about and move. If we are near a bathroom and have the time to void, the brain sends the message to this external sphincter to relax and allow emptying. If we are not near a bathroom or the time isn't appropriate, the brain sends a message down to this external sphincter to contract.

In addition, for bladder emptying to occur, two components of the bladder muscle itself must contract in synchronous fashion. The bladder is a smooth or nonvoluntary muscle that is under the control of the autonomic nervous system. The sympathetic nervous system supplies nerves to the bladder wall (6). When the wall contracts, the urine is pushed out of the bladder. The parasympathetic nervous system has nerves that run to the bladder neck (7), often called the internal sphincter. When this muscle contracts, it pulls the bladder neck open so that the urine can be pushed through. This is more graphically illustrated in figure 3.

All of the above must act in synchronization. In other words the external sphincter must be relaxed at the time that the bladder contracts and the bladder neck must also contract and open at the same time.

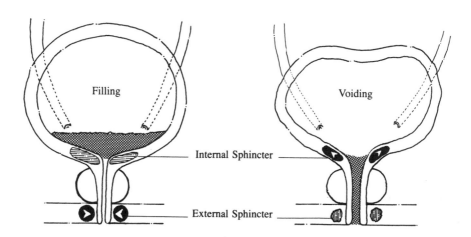

Fig. 3 Sphincter action during filling and voiding

PROBLEMS OF BLADDER CONTROL

The above system can fail at many points because of damage anywhere along the nervous system or because of structural changes. These problems can prevent emptying or cause frequent emptying out of control (incontinence), depending upon where the problem is.

If the external sphincter muscle is in spasm, such as can occur after a spinal-cord injury in which all voluntary muscles can be spastic, bladder emptying cannot occur no matter how hard the bladder contracts.

In males, the prostate surrounds the urethra between the external sphincter and the internal sphincter, or the bladder neck. If the prostate enlarges, as is quite common in older men, it prevents emptying of the bladder by actually mechanically blocking the urethra. This requires surgical treatment. Sometimes after surgery the bladder neck does not function properly, leading to incontinence. This will be discussed further in a later chapter.

Moreover, the angle of the bladder neck, or internal sphincter, can become abnormal, such as in women following multiple childbirths, or in the normal aging process. Or the external sphincter muscle itself may not contract readily. This causes a particular type of incontinence known as stress incontinence, meaning that urine will leak at the time of coughing, sneezing, or lifting heavy objects.

The nerves to the bladder may be directly damaged. This can occur in diabetes mellitus, spina bifida, or very low spinal-cord injuries in which the nerves are damaged after they leave the cord but are still inside the spinal canal. The bladder has no sensation and no ability to contract and so urine is retained. However, if the bladder becomes too full it will mechanically extend the bladder neck open and cause leakage of urine and incontinence.

Damage to the spinal cord, such as can occur in a spinal-cord injury or spina bifida, leaves the bladder functioning on its own. The nerves are able to transmit the signal to the spinal cord that the bladder is full. But the spinal cord cannot transmit the message to the brain.

Similarly in strokes, the bladder may be functioning on its own because the brain cannot receive the message. Multiple sclerosis can affect either the spinal cord or the brain and leave the bladder functioning independently.

What happens when the bladder functions on its own? The nerves transmit the full-bladder signal to the spinal cord. But the signal is blocked. The brain doesn't get the message. And so the brain cannot tell the external sphincter to tighten and prevent voiding. Therefore, the signal of distention (1) arrives at the spinal cord and immediately triggers the autonomic nervous system to send messages to contract the bladder (6) and open the bladder neck (7), causing bladder emptying.

The sensory pathways, either in the nerves from the bladder, or in the

43

nerve pathways in the spinal cord or brain, can alone be damaged. Such can occur in multiple sclerosis or occasionally in a stroke, and leads to the same sort of problem described above. The message cannot get through to the brain. The person has no idea that his bladder is about to contract and therefore no knowledge that he or she should contract the external sphincter. Bladder emptying occurs without the person's awareness.

PROBLEMS OF AN ABNORMAL BLADDER

With the previous understanding of normal and abnormal bladder emptying, or micturition, let's progress to some of the problems that can occur with an abnormal bladder mechanism and some of the things that you can do about it yourself. I do want to emphasize again that the purpose of this is to help a person understand his or her urinary system and be able to discuss the problem with a physician. There are many types of abnormal bladders, and there are different ways of dealing with each of these. It is not as simple as a bladder that won't empty and a bladder that empties too frequently. There are combinations of the two basic kinds of bladder dysfunction and your physician can best help you deal more directly with your own problem.

Incontinence is a serious problem, but unless it causes a skin breakdown that becomes infected, it is not necessarily life-threatening. Inability to empty the bladder, retaining urine, and a subsequent infection *are* life-threatening; therefore, one should be careful not to correct incontinence by methods that decrease the frequency or amount of urine.

EFFECTS OF RETAINED URINE

Inability to empty the bladder, or stasis of urine in the bladder leads to growth of bacteria in the bladder. Bacteria grow exponentially; that is, two become four, four become sixteen, sixteen become two hundred and fifty-six, so that growth starts off slow, but rapidly becomes very fast. Urine retained in the bladder is much like a stagnant pond covered with algae. Infected urine in the bladder is not life-threatening, but if not treated, the kidneys can become infected; and with repeated kidney infections, the kidneys slowly lose their ability to function, leading to a buildup of waste products in the body and ultimately to death.

Control of incontinence, then, should allow for frequent emptying to avoid stasis. The bladder is never emptied completely so there are always bacteria remaining in the urine once it is infected. It is important for you to know that the number of bacteria grows slowly at first, then rapidly. Figure 4 shows that in this particular hypothetical situation, by emptying the bladder

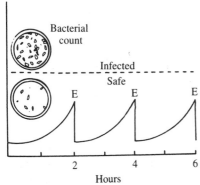

Fig. 4 The growth of bacteria related to emptying (E) of the bladder every two hours

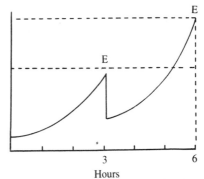

Fig. 5 The growth of bacteria related to emptying (E) of the bladder every three hours

at two hours the bacterial count is still low and the bacteria have not had a chance to multiply in their rapid phase and so the bacterial count in the urine remains low. Figure 5 shows that by waiting just an hour more, or three hours before emptying the bladder, the bacteria have begun to multiply rapidly and are more numerous. Thus when the bladder is emptied, even though the amount of urine is low, the number of bacteria is high and the urine can soon become significantly infected.

EFFECTS OF FLUID RESTRICTION

Since some urine, even if only an ounce or two, remains in the bladder, the effect of bacteria in the bladder is worse if not much urine is added per hour to dilute the number of bacteria. You can demonstrate this by taking a cup full of water and coloring it with a few drops of red food coloring. If you empty out one-quarter cup and replace it with one-quarter cup continually, you will slowly dilute out the red food coloring. If you dumped out three-quarters of a cup and replaced it with three-quarters of a cup, it would very rapidly dilute out the red food coloring. This is why it is important to maintain good fluid intake rather than avoid fluid intake to avoid incontinence.

The normal fluid intake is about 1,500 cc daily or six cups. Besides the effect on the urinary tract, there are effects on the whole body that arise from poor fluid intake or dehydration. As inadequate water can cause a plant to wither and die, so the lack of fluid can cause the electrolytes, the sodium and potassium in your body fluids, to get out of balance and this can cause weakness, a stupor, even cardiac irregularities and death. Also, severe lack of fluid itself can cause abrupt failure of the kidneys to function.

Other things cause decreased urine flow, besides lack of adequate intake or dehydration. Fluid is lost from the body in ways that doctors call insensible losses. The most obvious of these is fluid loss through excessive perspiration on a very hot day. Another is fluid loss through the lungs in mouth breathing when one has a stuffy nose from a cold. Sleep also decreases the rate of urine flow. Therefore, both for your general good health and for control of incontinence, frequent emptying is most important.

COPING WITH FREQUENCY

If your problem is frequent bladder emptying at inconvenient times, perhaps with an urge that allows you no time to get to the bathroom, or perhaps without an urge at all, then you should try to go more frequently than those occur, perhaps every one or two hours. This is particularly desirable if you have no feeling of a need to void. By scheduling a bathroom trip frequently, you may avoid the amount of bladder filling that would trigger an unfelt bladder response.

It is sometimes difficult to empty your bladder at specified times. There are techniques you can use to help. If you have difficulty starting to go because your bladder does not contract, and the bladder tends to retain urine, you can push on the lower abdomen over the bladder to help force urine out. This method is called crede. But if you are having trouble with urine going backward up the ureters, this may not be a good idea and you should discuss it with your physician before starting.

If your bladder empties too frequently, or, as we described, is a spastic bladder which empties on its own, you can trigger the spinal cord to respond by stroking the skin of your thighs, pinching or pulling pubic or thigh hairs, or at times digital stimulation of your rectum. Again, the best method for you can be discussed with your physician.

INFECTIONS

You should be aware of signs of infection. If your bladder is infected, it will be more irritable and you will have more difficulty with incontinence than is usual. Therefore, one of the signs of infection is increasing incontinence, or increased need to void frequently, or increased urgency—that is, difficulty making it to the bathroom after you feel the need to void. Foul-smelling urine, cloudy urine, and bloody urine are also signs of early infection and should signal you to call your physician before fever, chills, and kidney infection set in.

MEDICAL HELP FOR INCONTINENCE

Your doctor may prescribe an appropriate medication. If you can judge that the amount you empty is always very small, perhaps less than a cup

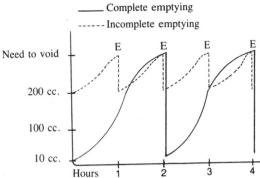

Fig. 6 The effect of incomplete emptying (E) of the bladder

as a rough estimate, a medication may be tried which may help relax the bladder as well as make it less irritable. Have a talk with your physician. He or she needs to check for complete emptying before starting such a medication.

Occasionally the bladder will not empty fully and because so much urine is left after voiding, the bladder rapidly fills up to the point where there is the need to void again. This is illustrated in figure 6. Again, it can be helped by medication, in this instance one that helps the bladder wall contract more and therefore helps emptying.

In either case, you should still be alert to voiding frequently and signs of infection.

On occasion, incontinence is more of a problem at night. If you void much urine in your sleep, your bladder should be emptied and there is nothing to do but awake and empty it. If the amount of urine is small, two possibilities may be occurring. One is that you may be awakening from some other cause and just be emptying your bladder "in case." You may be able to solve that problem by adjusting your environment to get rid of light or noise, or by taking a very mild medication that will cause drowsiness. It may also be that you need the medication described above to relax the bladder at nighttime only.

To help you live with incontinence, there are many products and devices that will be discussed at length in this book. One method of treating incontinence is an indwelling catheter into the bladder, often called a Foley catheter. This does control incontinence but leads to collection problems, a leg bag being required. Too, the Foley catheter is a foreign object in the bladder, which is always an infected object, even though it is sterile when inserted. Infection can lead to destruction of the bladder wall and to kidney infections and damage, even kidney failure.

I hope that this chapter has helped you understand the basic mechanics of the bladder so that you can discuss the particulars of your own case more knowledgeably with your physician.

5

Building Inner Confidence
Steven M. Tovian, Ph.D.
Ronald H. Rozensky, Ph.D

In Mesopotamia there lived a king and queen who ruled a small city-state. The king and queen prided themselves on their well-run, well-ordered land. A place for everything and everything in a place. They often traveled about their land talking with the people and enjoying nature. As time went on, however, they began to notice that not everything was as it could be. Occasionally leaves from trees would blow through the park instead of being immediately swept up. It even rained on days when royal picnics were scheduled. The king and queen became increasingly anxious about what they perceived as disorder.

Rather than continue to face these problems, they decided to retreat to the castle. They attended fewer and fewer gatherings. They spent less and less time walking in nature. The more time they spent away from their people, the more things seemed to stray from "a place for everything." The more this happened, the more they stayed in the castle, unable to face what they perceived as the growing disorder. The king and queen, dismayed by the turn of events, asked the three royal advisers for advice to remedy the problem.

The first said, "Your Majesties, this is indeed a problem. The land becomes more out of control as each day goes on, I suggest you stay in the castle, avoid the potential disarray. Be safe."

The second counseled, "You must go out amongst the people and present to them the reasons for control. Take with you the largest, strongest swordsman of the guard. If anything, man, woman, beast, or tree, challenges your order, let the swordsman strike."

The third adviser thought and said, "Let us consider the possibilities that you will encounter when you go forth amongst your people. What you see as disarray is finite. There are only so many trees, so many people, so many things they can all do or say. Let us plan a response to each. To each a response. Your order will show order. You can regain your control."

They did and it did happen.

Incontinence is life-disruptive medically, emotionally, and socially. Emotionally it can have an impact in immediately felt negative feelings, changes in self-image and self-confidence. Socially, shame, guilt, ridicule or isolation can be a factor. The major reason for focusing on the way you feel about incontinence is to help you understand, control, and plan for that wide range of possible reactions.

In our culture, the process of "toilet training" is important. Friends, doctors, and family ask, "Is he toilet-trained yet? What age? Can he make it through the night?" These can become pressures on young children which might eventually cause us all to be overly sensitive, even overreact, to incontinence.

Dr. Spock, author and pediatrician, writes in *Baby and Children*:

> Learning to use the toilet is an important forward step for children in several ways. They gain control of two apertures of the body that previously functioned automatically, and this gives them a lot of pride. . . They are accepting the first serious responsibility assigned by their parents. Successful cooperation on this major project will give parent and child a new confidence in each other. . . It's from their toilet training that children get some of their feelings that one way of doing things is right and another way is not; this helps them to develop a sense of obligation, to become systematic people. So toilet training plays a part in the formation of children's character and in building the basic trust between them and their parents.

Psychoanalyst Erik Erikson, on discussing childhood bowel and bladder training, writes that the child experiences a "premium of satisfaction over a major job well done" with increased control. The developing child, he says, learns a sense of autonomous will as it learns to "hold on" or "let go." With this comes a sense of self-control without loss of self-esteem. But a loss of self-control leads to self-doubt and shame. Shame, according to Erikson, is an early emotion that "exploits the increased sense of being small" or childlike.

From these discussions of the importance of bladder control, we can see why people have little tolerance for, and even discomfort with, incontinence. The emotions triggered by incontinence can cause either the outside observer or the individual with the problem to feel small or childlike, shamed, lacking in self-control, and then self-doubt. From the interviews in Chapter 2, we find that the concept of self-control and the feelings associated with loss of control are very important among incontinent people. Society is equally uncomfortable with the apparent helplessness of incontinent persons.

Control of your emotional response to incontinence occurs at two levels. First, awareness of your own internal response to the problem, and second, managing your reaction to the social reaction to you and your problem.

PSYCHOSOCIAL PROBLEMS AND INCONTINENCE

Most of the research written on incontinence offers a few general statements about what a distressing condition it is. There may be talk by authors of the social problems occurring with incontinence and how embarrassing it is to be wet or soiled, but little attempt has been made to look at how each person feels about his or her condition and copes with it. Social taboos may inhibit patients from more open discussions. Incontinence often affects those groups least able to demand services (elderly, physically handicapped).

Lack of professional interest may be supported by old beliefs that incontinence is used solely by the patient for getting physical care and social attention, dramatizing emotions such as depression or immaturity, and avoiding certain activities in daily life. However, a nurse, C. Norton, gave a detailed questionnaire to fifty-five women suffering from incontinence at a urology clinic in Great Britain. She asked these women questions about the psychological and social effects of being incontinent. The results from this survey offer an important scientific starting point for understanding the incontinent. This study revealed that the amount of incontinence or leakage had nothing to do with the degree of emotional distress experienced by the women. The range of their difficulties with themselves and others, and their severity, had nothing to do with age, length of time being incontinent, or the cause of incontinence. Each person's reactions were individual in nature. Each individual perceives his or her incontinence differently and will react with varying degrees of emotional distress.

IDENTIFYING CAUSES OF STRESS

Patients in the study reported a range of feelings, including depression, irritability, anxiety, worry, frustration, and anger in response to their incontinence. Others reported feeling constantly toilet-centered in their thoughts and activities. In one person, incontinence was the main underlying cause of a near "nervous breakdown," showing itself in obsessional anxiety over hygiene. Anxiety, fear, and never being able to relax and forget the problem were recurrent comments from the women in the study—"I am continually worried about being wet"; "I feel very afraid of going out"; "My leakage problem . . . makes me tense and irritable"; "I get panicky when I cannot reach a toilet"; "I am so irritable that I hate myself."

In other areas, incontinence has been found to reduce the individual's ability to undertake any form of physical exercise. Many patients give up sports, dancing, jogging, and long walks. Problems in performing daily chores arise especially because of leakage occurring when lifting anything heavy. Some women in the study reported repeated toilet visits interrupting outings, and needing to be able to stop at places with known and easily accessible toilet facilities. "I am frightened to venture too far from home," one woman wrote, and another said, "Shopping must be done in the shortest of time."

Social life of the incontinent is severely inhibited or reduced. Fear of disasters in social situations makes people alter their lifestyle to avoid potential problems. Being self-conscious at social functions is a common occurrence. Women reported that they worried about leakage when in the company of others, so they avoided getting physically close to people in case of offending others. Embarrassment and choosing social withdrawal are common.

The relationship with the family was the least negatively affected area in Norton's study. Many patients praised their families for tolerance and understanding. In one case, a patient's incontinence brought family members closer together, and in another case, support was gained from the family's sense of humor. Here the patient's children adopted names like Mom's Plumber's Pack for her ever present bag of clothes and pads. However, those patients with unsupportive families felt extremely threatened and vulnerable. One woman told of her eleven-year-old daughter who would often say aloud, "Mommy, you smell bad!" Others who had hidden the problem from family had constant fear it would be discovered. They sat on opposite sides of the room so their children would not notice leakage or odor. On especially bad days when some patients were particularly irritable, their children and spouses were frequent targets of their displaced anger.

In two cases from the study, incontinence was cited as the primary cause for divorce. Incontinence also led to ceasing sexual intercourse for several women while others were very embarrassed by leakage during intercourse. There were others who feared cystitis as a result of bladder problems during sexual relations. Many women simply felt unattractive wearing pads in bed, or were annoyed by repeated interruptions during intercourse to go to the toilet. Also feeling "dirty and smelly" from incontinence resulted in a decrease in lovemaking.

Several patients lost their jobs as a result of their incontinence or had to change their positions because of restrictions on activities. For some women fear of odor and/or leakage impaired work concentration, especially at meetings.

Many women felt obliged to wear old or unattractive clothing for ease of washing or to prevent stains from showing. Tight clothes were avoided because pads might show. Reactions to wearing trousers varied: some said they would never wear them, others said they could not wear anything else. Those who wore a dress most often wore plastic pants as well. Many women felt unattractive because they were forced to wear unbecoming clothing.

51

The women often feared they smelled of urine and avoided becoming physically close to others. Such women called themselves "antisocial" or "segregated" when in public. We live in a society that has tabooed normal body odors; we use deodorants and mouthwashes to avoid being offensive. Whether the women's fear was realistic or not, it altered their lifestyle by avoiding groups, constantly wondering if people noticed the odor, and finally deciding it was far easier being alone.

Like smell, embarrassment restricted the activities of many patients. The constant anxiety and inability to forget about leakage for any length of time seemed to depress them. One woman had a constant nightmare of being at the end of a long line to a public toilet when she needed it. Embarrassment was caused not only by incontinence but also by urinary frequency. One woman, for example, was unable to go to the theater because of having to excuse herself time after time.

WHAT ARE THE WORST PROBLEMS

When questioned about the worst effect of leakage or incontinence on their lives, many in the Norton study felt it was the shame they experienced. Such a feeling contributes to a general lack of self-confidence in a person because if one is not in control of one's own body, what else is beyond one's ability to control or cope with? One woman imagined herself standing in a pool of water with a group of friends laughing at her.

Others felt that relentless and always present anxiety was the worst effect of incontinence. A lack of peace of mind and fear of the future dominated many patients' thoughts. Many thought being incontinent was far worse than having leakage because leakage meant smaller amounts whereas incontinence meant total loss of control. Younger patients feared that their leakage would become total incontinence as they grew old.

Others were most bothered by embarrassment from reactions of other people to their incontinence, especially spouses and children. These women found explaining their condition to their children most stressful and others readily cited incontinence as a major cause of marital problems. For these women, wearing wet, perhaps smelly pads, and the inconvenience, when in public, of constantly having to find public restrooms were acutely embarrassing. Others saw a specific restriction such as being "unable to go on a vacation" as the worst effect. Some summed it all up this way: "Incontinence has an effect on everything I do or wish to do." One woman saw it as a major problem because incontinence had made her "virtually housebound."

WHAT IS COPING?

From this discussion of identifying social and emotional problems and incontinence, let us now discuss how one copes with the problem. *Coping* is a word often used when talking about reactions to illness, disability, crisis, or even natural disasters like floods and severe storms. Coping describes what one does about a problem to bring about relief, calm, emotional balance, or the feelings that were present before the problem began. This description has three important parts. First, there is a recognized problem from which one seeks relief. Second, what one does or does not do about that problem suggests something about how one copes. Third, there is some result or outcome which may or may not be effective, and which may achieve only short-term relief.

Coping may be seen either as your action or behavior, or as your way to manage, master, tolerate, reduce, or minimize demands and conflicts coming from the outside world, or even from within yourself which tax or drain your resources. Coping is a series of related steps or strategies and not a single set of independent actions. Coping does not mean merely feeling better or less troubled by a problem. It is also important to know that what one does or did added to the relief or solving of the problem. This fosters a sense of increased control.

Coping is something we do every day. We hardly notice this unless a problem continues and we start to feel increasing emotional distress. Look for some unresolved problem whenever emotional distress occurs. For example, try to recall an occasion in the past month when you felt—shame, humiliation, depression, annoyance, anger, resentment, tension, helplessness, sorrow, guilt, embarrassment, discouragement, fear.

These feelings, largely unwelcome, can be called emotional distress. Emotional distress that occurs over and over may suggest unresolved past or present problems. Some of these feelings will often go away on their own; others need to be coped with using one strategy or another.

To know more about coping with your incontinence, ask yourself these questions:

1. What problems do you see your incontinence creating?
2. When faced with a problem you must do something about, what happens? What do you do? How do you feel? How often does it occur?
3. How does it usually work out?
4. To whom do you turn if you need help?

5. What kinds of situations usually cause you distress?
6. How has your incontinence affected people closest to you?

COPING STRATEGIES

The goals of any coping strategy include preserving your emotional balance by managing the emotional distress caused by incontinence; preserving a satisfactory self-image and maintaining a sense of competence and mastery despite your incontinence; preserving your relationships with family and friends; and dealing with any special-treatment procedures which may be related to the incontinence.

What are the strategies or things people do to cope with problems? Often people use more than one strategy, and each strategy is not necessarily good or bad. Coping is good provided the approach you use is socially sanctioned or not reckless or harmful to oneself or others. It is important to understand exactly what your problem is if you hope to deal with it effectively. Following is a list of some coping strategies:

1. Seeking more information.
2. Talking with others who have a similar problem.
3. Laughing and making light of the problem.
4. Trying to forget or deny.
5. Doing other things for distraction.
6. Taking firm action based on what you know about a problem.
7. Accepting or finding something favorable about a problem situation.
8. Submitting passively to the inevitable.
9. Doing something reckless or impulsive.
10. Withdrawing into isolation.
11. Blaming someone or something.
12. Seeking direction and doing what you're told.
13. Blaming yourself.
14. Considering feasible alternatives in a future problem situation.

EFFECTIVE STRATEGIES

There is no secret formula for good coping that fits everyone with incontinence. Coping is a skill that calls upon other skills best suited to the occasion. If one action better prepares a person for the next problem, then whatever works best is best for that person. The important issues in any coping strategy are: What are the results? And has emotional distress been reduced?

If coping is a skill, then it can be learned using the characteristics of good copers. Research has found that good copers with other serious chronic illnesses such as diabetes and cancer seem to follow these guidelines:

1. Do not deny too often, or too long.
2. Confront reality and take appropriate action.
3. Focus on solutions to problems.
4. Consider alternatives to problems—be flexible.
5. Maintain open, honest, mutual communication with others important to you.
6. Seek and use constructive outside help.
7. Accept support offered, but seek independence whenever possible.
8. Keep up morale through self-reliance.
9. Develop a good self-concept, which is an important solution to any problem.

Good copers know the difference between being hopeless and powerless on one hand, and active and assertive on the other. Poor copers are rigid, overly compliant, and lack self-assertion. In fact, the difference between good copers and poor copers is the difference between resourcefulness and rigidity; between constructive optimism and pessimism where one expects a repeat of earlier defeats. Good copers confront problems, do what they can to solve them and reduce distress, and call upon available supports, including their own inner resources. They demand and yield selectively, anticipating blunt realities, and knowing that not every problem can be solved every time. Nevertheless, problems can be solved more through awareness and acceptance than by disavowal, avoidance, and denial. Poor copers also mistake bravado, or a habit of saying "I can do it myself," for independence. It takes more courage to recognize a problem and accept help than to strive for unrealistic independence. Indeed, poor copers usually deny a great deal despite the existence of real problems, call on wishful thinking, or use overly passive approaches waiting for something to be done for them by others.

SUMMARY

Clearly, incontinence has serious emotional and social effects upon people, thus reducing the quality of their life. One can only speculate how it affects people when additional disabilities and medical problems are present. Emotional and social problems related to incontinence are summarized below, based upon viewing these problems according to the following attributes: behavior (activities); affect (emotions or feelings); sensations (physical experiences); imagery (picturing scenes in one's mind); and cognition (thoughts or self-statements). The first letter of each attribute spells BASIC; the acronym represents a convenient method of assessing the many ways incontinence may result in psychological problems. This method of assessment was developed more fully by psychologist Dr. A. Lazarus, and when applied to incontinence such an analysis may look like this:

BEHAVIOR (ACTIVITIES)

1. Social withdrawal and isolation
2. Difficulty doing activities of daily living
3. Job change or loss of job
4. Sexual dysfunction
5. Wearing unattractive clothing

AFFECT (EMOTIONS OR FEELINGS)

1. Shame or embarrassment
2. Depression
3. Irritability or anger
4. Anxiety, worry, tension
5. Frustration
6. Vulnerability

SENSATIONS (PHYSICAL EXPERIENCES)

1. Odor
2. Tenseness in various muscles throughout the body.

IMAGERY (PICTURING SCENES IN ONE'S MIND)

1. Standing in a pool of water with friends laughing at me.
2. Having to explain to my children that I wet myself and my bed just like an infant.
3. Being in a store with no public restroom available.
4. Finding a public restroom but having to wait in a long line.
5. Going to a movie but having to leave my seat repeatedly to go to the restroom.

6. Explaining to my spouse that I must use pads in bed during intercourse because of leakage.
7. People moving away from me on a bus because of odor.

COGNITION (THOUGHTS OR SELF-STATEMENTS)

1. I must be near a toilet at all times or I will panic.
2. I must smell terrible and be soiled.
3. I am afraid to go out in public.
4. I hate myself and lack confidence.
5. I am ugly.
6. If I cannot control this part of my body, what will be next?
7. I am helpless and hopeless.

We have discussed coping and how it applies to incontinence. In the next chapter, we will talk about specific ways to deal with these psychosocial problems, and supply ideas for handling incontinence in social situations. You may wish to read further on some of the issues discussed in this chapter. We recommend the following books or articles:

1. Lazarus, A. *The Practice of Multi-Modal Therapy*. New York: McGraw-Hill, 1981.
2. Norton, C. The Effects of Urinary Incontinence in Women. *Int. Rehab. Med.* 4:9–14. 1982.
3. Weisman, A. *Coping with Cancer*. New York: McGraw-Hill, 1979.

6

Strategies for a Full Life

Ronald H. Rozensky, Ph.D.
Steven M. Tovian, Ph.D.

If helplessness is the precursor to depression, then hopelessness is the invitation to the incontinent person to stay home. If shame is the lock on the door, then control is the key.

The way out is to change. To change is to gain control over your response to the world about you. To feel in control, to be in control, to focus on ways to create that sense of control you are looking for is to gain mastery over those social, emotional, personal restrictions that, until now, you have felt imprisoned you. To have a repertoire, a list of options to cope with the problems of incontinence, will provide for you a sense of freedom, a sense of preparedness to cope with your own feelings and those of others.

Given the spectrum of emotional responses to incontinence discussed above, and with the understanding of the foundational issue of control and self-esteem, you will find in this chapter a variety of self-change methods designed to enhance control of your emotional response to incontinence.

STRATEGIES FOR CHANGE

We have identified the psychological problems that are a result of incontinence. In the following sections we will briefly describe five specific strategies to handle your problems. These are perhaps the most important of the many ways of coping emotionally with incontinence. The strategies are listed corresponding to the specific problem that emerges in table 1. A more detailed discussion of these techniques is found in a book *The Relaxation and Stress Reduction Workbook* by Martha Davis, Elizabeth R. Eshelman, and Mathew McKay, (New Harbinger Publications, 1980).

PROGRESSIVE RELAXATION

You cannot have feelings of warm well-being in your body and at the same time experience psychological stress. Progressive relaxation of your muscles reduces tension, anxiety, insomnia, and depression. Most people do not realize when they are chronically tense. Progressive relaxation provides a way of identifying particular muscles and muscle groups and telling the difference between tension and relaxation. The body responds to anxiety-provoking thoughts and events with muscle tension. The tension, in turn, increases the person's anxiety. Deep muscle relaxation reduces tension and helps rid you of anxiety. The habit of responding with one blocks the habit of responding with the other. Four major muscle groups are covered:

1. Hands, forearms, and biceps.
2. Head, face, neck and shoulders, including forehead, nose, eyes, jaws, and lips.
3. Chest, stomach, and lower back.
4. Thighs, buttocks, calves and feet.

Progressive relaxation can be practiced lying down or in a chair with your head supported. Each muscle from each group is tensed from five to seven seconds and then relaxed for twenty to thirty seconds. This procedure is repeated at least once. If an area remains tense, you can practice up to five times. You may also find it useful to say or think the following when untensing:

Let go of the tension.
Throw away the tension; I am feeling calm and rested.
Relax and smooth out the muscles.
Let the tension dissolve away.

Once the procedure is familiar enough to be remembered, you may wish to keep your eyes closed and focus attention on just one muscle group at a time. The instructions for progressive relaxation are divided into two sections. The first part, which you may wish to tape and replay when practicing, will familiarize you with the muscles in your body which are most commonly tense. This procedure takes fifteen to twenty minutes, needs to be practiced once or twice per day, and takes about two weeks of practice to master. The second section shortens the procedure after the first part is mastered and involves simultaneously tensing and relaxing many muscles so that deep muscle relaxation can be achieved in a very brief period.

Some people begin their relaxation exercises with deep breathing exercises:

1. Inhaling a complete natural breath.
2. Holding this breath for a few seconds.
3. Exhaling a little air with force through a small hole between your lips as though you were blowing through a straw. Stop exhaling for a moment and then blow out a bit more air. Repeat this until all the air is exhaled in small puffs.

REFUTING IRRATIONAL IDEAS

You constantly engage in self-talk, your internal thought language, sometimes called cognition. These are the sentences with which you describe and interpret the world. If the self-talk is accurate and in touch with reality, you function well. If it is irrational and untrue, then you experience anxiety, depression, and emotional disturbance. This sentence is an example of irrational self-talk leading to the feeling of hopelessness: "I can't bear to be alone." No physically stable person has ever died merely from being alone. Being alone may be uncomfortable, undesirable, and frustrating, but you can live with it, live through it, and use options to change it.

Another example of irrational self-talk: "I must never have an accident in public. If I do, I'm a failure as a person." The words "must never" allow no possibility of flaw. Should the inevitable occur, you label yourself rotten—all on the basis of a single incident.

Irrational ideas may be based on outright misperceptions or perfectionistic shoulds, oughts, and musts. Inaccurate self-talk such as "How terrible to be rejected" is fear-producing in comparison with "I find it unpleasant, and momentarily awkward and regrettable when I am rejected."

Albert Ellis, a psychologist, developed a system to attack irrational ideas or beliefs and replace them with realistic statements about the world. His basic notion is that emotions have nothing to do with actual events. In between the event and the emotion is realistic or unrealistic self-talk. It is the self-talk that produces the emotions. Your own thoughts, directed and controlled by you, are what create anxiety, anger, and depression. The following diagram explains how it works:

Events in
Environment

Perceptions &
Cognitions

Interpretation
Self-Talk
Which Can Be
Irrational

Emotions &
Behavior

Feedback Loop

At the root of all irrational thinking is the assumption that things are done to you. Nothing is done to you. Events happen in the world. You experience those events (A), engage in self-talk (B), and then experience an emotion (C), resulting from the self-talk. A does not cause C; B causes C. If your self-talk is irrational and unrealistic, you create unpleasant emotions.

Two common forms of irrational self-talk are statements that "catastrophize" and "absolutize." You catastrophize by making terrible, nightmarish interpretations of your experience. A momentary leakage will become a pool of urine. The emotions that follow catastrophizing self-talk tend to be awful, for you are responding to that very description of the event.

Irrational self-statements that "absolutize" often include words like *should, must, ought, always, never.* Events have to be a certain way, or you have to be a certain way. Any deviation from that particular value or standard is bad. The person who fails to live up to the standard is bad. In fact, it is the standard that is bad, because it is irrational.

Dr. Ellis has suggested ten irrational ideas. Think how they can be related to incontinence problems.

- I must have love and approval from peers, family, and friends.
- It is horrible when people or things are not the way I'd like them to be.
- I should fear anything that is unknown or uncertain.
- It is easier to avoid than face life's difficulties.
- You need something other or stronger or greater than yourself to rely on.
- The past determines the present.
- Happiness can be achieved by passivity.
- You are helpless and have no control over what you feel, experience, or do.
- When people disapprove of you, it means you are wrong or bad.
- You shouldn't have to feel pain; you are entitled to a good life.

Much of the difficulty in uncovering irrational self-talk results from the speed in which thoughts occur. Self-talk has a reflexive, automatic quality. However, once thoughts are slowed down, you can assess their rationality and impact.

Below are five steps (A through E) to disputing and eliminating irrational ideas. Start by selecting a situation that consistently generates disturbing emotions in you.

A. Write down the facts of the events as they occurred.
B. Write down your self-talk about the event.

C. Focus on your emotional response (anger, depression, worthlessness, fear, etc.).

D. Dispute and change the irrational self-talk.

1. Select the irrational idea you wish to change (e.g., *"It is not fair that I have to suffer with incontinence"*).

2. Is there any rational support for this idea? (The problem must be endured and dealt with because it happened. It happened because all conditions existed necessary to make it happen.)

3. What evidence exists for the falseness of this idea that I had to suffer with incontinence? (There is no guarantee that says I should not have pain or problems through incontinence— no laws of the universe. I can experience any problem for which the necessary conditions exist. Life is not fair. Life is a sequence of events, some of which are inconvenient and painful. If problems occur, it is up to me to solve them. No one is special. Some go through life with relatively fewer problems than I. This probably traces to luck or decisions I have made that contributed to the necessary conditions for my problems. Just because I am incontinent does not mean I have to suffer. I can take pride in the challenge of a creative solution. This may be an opportunity to increase my self-esteem.)

4. Does any evidence exist for the truth of this irrational idea? (No, my suffering could stem from self-talk or how I have interpreted my incontinence. I have convinced myself I should be unhappy.)

5. Sometimes focusing on the "worst" alternative helps you plan ahead. (I could be deprived as a result of incontinence of various pleasures while I deal with the incontinence. I might feel inconvenienced. I might never solve the problem and accept the consequences. Others may not approve of how I am behaving and I could be rejected.)

6. Is there anything positive that you can find in this experience? (From incontinence, I might learn to tolerate frustration better or improve my coping skills.)

E. Substitute alternative self-talk now that you have examined the irrational idea and compared it with rational thinking. (I can accept painful situations when they arise from my incontinence. Facing problems from incontinence is more adaptive than resenting it or running away from it. I feel what I think. At worst, with incontinence I will experience inconvenience, regret, and annoyance— not anxiety, depression, and rage.)

ASSERTIVENESS TRAINING

Assertiveness training can reduce anxiety and depression by teaching you to stand up for your legitimate rights without bullying others (aggression) or letting them bully you (passivity). Assertiveness means expressing personal rights and feelings. You are assertive when you stand up for your rights in such a way that the rights of others are not violated. Beyond merely demanding your rights in situations, you can express your personal rights spontaneously, you can ask for clarification, you can talk about yourself without being self-conscious, you can disagree with someone openly, and you can say no when you are an assertive person. You can also be more relaxed in interpersonal situations. Some people think that assertiveness turns nice people into terrible, mean complainers or manipulators. Not true. It is your right to protect yourself when something seems unfair. You are the one who best knows your discomfort and your needs.

Several months of step-by-step work are often necessary for some individuals to learn assertiveness training. Such a detailed explanation is beyond the scope of this chapter. For that reason a brief outline of assertiveness training is presented here with references for more comprehensive training included at the end of this chapter.

When learning assertiveness training, one must be aware of those legitimate rights he or she has as an adult individual. Here is a partial list of those legitimate rights taken from the *Relaxation and Stress Reduction Workbook.*

- You have the right, at times, to put yourself first.
- You have the right to make mistakes.
- You have the right to be the final judge of your feelings.
- You have the right to have your own opinions.
- You have the right to change your mind or decide on a different course of action.
- You have a right to protest unfair treatment.
- You have a right to ask for clarification.
- You have a right to negotiate for change.
- You have a right to ask for help or emotional support.
- You have a right to say no.
- You have a right not to have to justify yourself to others.
- You have a right not to take responsibility for someone else's problem.
- You have a right not to have to anticipate other's needs and wishes.
- You have a right to choose not to respond to people's questions.

Once these legitimate rights are understood and accepted, it is important to identify those specific situations in which you want to be more effective. Ask yourself:

- Who are the persons involved?
- When does the situation take place?
- What bothers you?
- How do you deal with the situation and your feelings?
- What do you fear will take place if you are assertive?
- What are your goals?

Summarizing the steps involved in responding in an assertive manner, you would:

1. Look at your rights and ask what you want and feel about the specific situation.
2. Let go of blame, the desire to hurt others, and self-pity.
3. Describe your feelings with "I messages." "I messages" express your feelings without evaluating or blaming others. Rather than say, "You hurt me," the "I message" would be simply, "I feel hurt." "I messages" connect your feelings with the specific behavior of the other person. "I felt hurt when you laughed at me" is far better than "I felt hurt because you were inconsiderate and cruel."
4. Express your request in one or two easy-to-understand sentences. Be specific, maintain direct eye-contact, erect body posture. Speak clearly and firmly; don't yell, whine, or apologize (unless you're wrong).
5. Reinforce the possibility of getting what you want by stating the positive consequences should the other person cooperate with you. If necessary, state the consequences for failure to cooperate.

Consider the problem of loneliness and isolation using assertiveness skills. You can consider techniques for getting out of the house as a "ladder to more productive living." The first letters in the following six steps for assertiveness spell *ladder*. Use this device to recall the steps toward assertive behavior.

1. Look at your rights, what you want, what you need, and your feelings about the situation. For example, "It is vital for me to go out and socialize with my wife in spite of my incontinence and her discomfort about a possible accident."
2. Arrange a time and place to work on this problem. "I will ask her

to discuss it after dinner Friday night, or as soon afterward as possible."

3. *D*efine the problem. "She seems so uncomfortable when we've gone out for fear of my having an accident. We haven't gone out for months now."
4. *D*escribe your feelings. "I feel frustrated that she feels embarrassed. I also feel hurt that she won't talk about the problem. Besides, I'm feeling depressed about being a prisoner in my own home."
5. *E*xpress your request. To the wife: "I'd like to go out."
6. *R*einforce the possibility of getting what you want by stating positive consequences should the other person cooperate with you. "I have taken precautions should an accident occur. I don't want to feel embarrassed, but staying home all the time just isn't good for our relationship. I can cope with this but I want your support as well."

THOUGHT STOPPING

Thought stopping can help you overcome the nagging worry and doubt that stand in the way of relaxation. Repetitive and intrusive trains of thought, or obsessions, are often unrealistic, unproductive, and anxiety-provoking. Obsessions may take the form of self-doubt: "Because of my incontinence, I'll never go back to work." Obsessions may also take the form of fear: "I wonder if I'll have an accident in public tonight at the party."

Thought stopping involves concentrating on the unwanted thoughts and, after a brief time, suddenly stopping and emptying your mind. The command "stop" is generally said to oneself and used to interrupt the unpleasant thoughts. It serves as a punishment, and any behavior that is constantly punished is likely to be reduced or inhibited. The command "stop" also acts as a distractor, and the self-instruction is incompatible with the obsessive thought. Thought stopping is an assertive response and can be followed by thought substitutions of reassuring or self-accepting statements. Negative and frightening thoughts come before negative and frightening emotions. If the thoughts can be controlled, overall stress can be significantly reduced.

Example: "Because of my incontinence, I must have a terrible odor— Stop! I have taken steps to control any potential odors and if one should arise, I will be the first to notice and can take steps to correct any problem."

COPING-SKILLS TRAINING

Coping-skills training teaches you to relax away anxiety and stress. It provides a greater ability for self-control in the particular situations that you find anxiety-provoking. It is not necessary, just because you are in a stressful situation, to feel nervous and upset. You have merely learned to react that way.

First, coping-skills training involves identifying those situations which cause you the most stress.

Second, it involves using the techniques of progressive relaxation training (discussed earlier) to relax and let go of any physical tension.

Last, coping-skills training involves creating a personal group of stress coping remarks. These will be used to get you through the periods when you are saying to yourself, I can't do this . . . I'm not strong enough. . .

The training simply involves rehearsal in imagination for the real-life events you find distressing. You learn to relax in the imagined scenes, and are thereafter prepared to relax tension away when under fire. Eventually, self-relaxation procedures and stress coping thoughts become automatic in any stressful situation.

For example, let us consider a method for coping with an "accident" of incontinence in public as an excellent example of coping-skills training.

METHOD FOR COPING WITH AN ACCIDENT

The very use of the term *accident* to describe what happens to an incontinent person when he "accidentally" voids in a public setting suggests the full range of possible emotional responses discussed so far. One dictionary definition of *accident* is an "unforeseen or unplanned event"; another, something "resulting from carelessness, unawareness, ignorance. . ." Further definitions suggest that it the accident we are discussing is indeed no one's fault, does not arise from carelessness, and, though unplanned, is not unforeseen.

Sadly, it is often a matter of not *if* but *when* an accident will happen. Planning your coping strategy for accidents makes the unplanned planned, the unforeseen a foreseen reality. Thus, we can manage the severity of an emotional response to the situation. If shame is a common response, then PRIDE, *p*lanned *r*espose for *i*ndividually *d*ealing with your *e*motions, is the opposite. You no longer have accidents; instead, because of your medical condition, you will at times void when you don't want to and you will create for yourself a PRIDEful response to that complex problem. Let's follow the BASIC solution.

B—BEHAVIOR

1. Know all routes to the bathroom.
2. Bring extra clothing in a stylish bag.

3. Use assertive responses in knowing what to say:
   a. You don't have to tell others anything, if you so desire.
   b. You can tell others in advance of a possible accident to avoid surprises.

A—AFFECT (Emotions)

1. How did you feel in the same situation in the past?
2. How would you like to feel? Identify that feeling.

S—SENSATIONS (Physical Feelings)

1. Use relaxation training from all your practice.

I—IMAGERY

1. See yourself prepared in the evident of an accident. No longer "accident-prone" in response to your incontinence.
2. Picture yourself emotionally calm, relaxed, confident in handling the situation.

C—COGNITION (Thoughts)

1. "I'm going to be all right."
   "It's easier once I get started."
   "There's nothing to worry about."
   "It cannot destroy me."
   "If I don't think of fear, I won't be afraid."
   "I can only do my best."
   "I can do this."

   "I can take care of myself. I'm prepared."
   "I have a specific plan for solving this."
   "I am afraid because I decided to be. I can decide not to be."

   "Relax now!"
   "This too shall end."
   "I've survived this, this and worse before."
   "Concentrate on deep breathing."

   "I did it!"
   "I did well."
   "It is possible not to be scared. Stop thinking I'm scared."
   "It is easier to turn off worry."

You will notice an emphasis on thoughts or cognitions in coping-skills training. This is important because your interpretations of the situation, predictions, and self-evaluations are what create emotions. If you say to yourself, it's too much for me to handle being in public, then the emotional response will be fear. If your self-statement is, those people will just laugh at me, then your emotional response will be more fear or anger.

If you say to yourself, I'm going to fail, then your body's response may be a knot in your stomach. Noticing this unpleasant physical reaction, you might think, I'm panicking, I can't go on; I must go home. These self-statements in turn increase your body's anxiety responses and can cause you to make poor decisions. The feedback loop from thoughts to physical reactions to behavioral choices to more negative thoughts can continue unbroken into a state of chronic anxiety.

The more attention you give to your thoughts and self-statements, the quicker you'll achieve relief from anxiety. Your thoughts don't have to intensify fear. Instead, they can act to calm you and push away panic.

Your most successful stress coping thoughts are worth writing down. Memorize a number of them for each stage in coping: preparation for stress; facing the challenge; noticing any fear; and self-reward. Make the coping statements meaningful to you and change them if they lose their impact.

Some people, especially when depressed, are afraid to congratulate them- selves for any achievement. They harbor the belief that self-praise causes disaster. What this really means is that something else, such as fate or luck, is also given credit for their successes. Taking credit for coping with in- continence means that you are responsible for how things turn out, and you have the power to limit painful emotions and problematic behavior.

WHEN THINGS DON'T COME EASY

At some point, you may have difficulty in exchanging old habits for new, more rewarding ones. Change might not always come easy—you may feel stuck in your old nonrewarding ways— but continue to try to change. Patience, persistence, and time are the only things needed.

If you continue to have difficulty starting more positive changes, consider the following roadblocks to change. A surprising number of people are attached to their problems related to incontinence, problems which serve a definite purpose. For example, a woman's leakage may get her out of sexual situations she may want to avoid, without having to take responsibility for disappointing or confronting her spouse. You can find out whether problems related to your incontinence rescue you from more unpleasant experiences by keeping a log of when such problems involving incontinence arise and the activities (or would-be activities) pertaining to them. If you suspect that additional problems connected with your incontinence provide you "secondary gain" in this manner, review the section in this chapter on assertiveness training. It should provide you with the incentive and the tools to be more direct in saying no.

Your feelings about your incontinence may lie buried. For example, you may be angry with your family but you do not share this fact with them. The people around you are apt to be aware that you are withholding stressful feelings and that something is wrong. Nevertheless, they cannot read your mind, and are unlikely to come to your rescue. You know best what you need. Letting others know your feelings and what you want opens the way to engaging them in helping you make a change.

Your symptoms may be a way of getting taken care of when you feel that you cannot directly ask for help or consideration. Many of us have learned since childhood that illness, sickness, and disability are often the only means of gaining support and physical comfort from others.

It is possible that your reactions to incontinence are patterned after the reactions of an important person in your life (mother or father) to illness or disability. You often develop the emotional responses of such a person as part of your identification with that one. Characteristic ways of reacting to illness and stress are generally learned, so ask yourself who in your family shares similar ways of reacting. It is often easier to realize how that one is not dealing effectively with illness or stress than to realize it in yourself. The next step is to observe and see if the same is true of you.

Finally, there are limits to self-modification. If you continue to have difficulty developing new, more rewarding ways of coping, consider consulting a professional. Professional help can introduce new situations that encourage the development of new behavior and emotions. Choosing a professional helper can seem a difficult task. We recommend a licensed clinical or counseling psychologist, psychiatrist, or social worker knowledgeable and experienced in medical psychology and, if possible, incontinence. Make inquiries about such professionals among fellow patients; consult your medical doctors, university hospital, or medical center for recommendations of various professionals or even groups available dealing with incontinence or emotional reactions to illness and disability.

In the end, don't give up. Your ability to increase control and make positive changes in coping with incontinence is a tremendous power. Persistence and determination are important parts in developing this power.

RECOMMENDED READING

If you're interested in reading further on the specific strategies for change discussed in this chapter, we recommend:

1. Progressive Relaxation
   Jacobsen, E. *Progressive Relaxation*. Chicago: University of Chicago Press, Midway Press, 1974.
2. Refuting Irrational Ideas
   Ellis, A. *A New Guide to Rational Living*. North Hollywood, Calif.: Wilshire Books, 1975.
   Goodman, D. S. *Emotional Well-Being Through Rational Behavior Training*. Springfield, Ill.: Charles C. Thomas, 1974.
3. Assertiveness Training
   Alberti, R. E., and Emmons, M. *Your Perfect Right*. San Luis Obispo, Calif.: Impact Press, 1974.
   Fensterheim, H. *Don't Say Yes When You Want to Say No*. New York: D. McKay, 1975.
   Smith, M. J. *When I Say No, I Feel Guilty*. New York: Dial Press, 1975.
   Coping-Skills Training
4. Meichenbaum, D. "Self-Instructional Methods." In *Helping People Change*, edited by F. K. Kaufner and A. P. Goldstein. New York: Pergamon Press, 1974.

7

Try Humor for a Change

Cheryle Gartley and Henry Holden

We are all here for a spell—
Get all the good laughs you can.
—Will Rogers

Editor's note: Some of you may think we should apologize for finding humor in incontinence. There was a time, not long ago in fact, when I would have wholeheartedly agreed. But no longer. I have discovered that somewhere, hidden in any of the circumstances life hands to us, is a little bit of fun. Why not go looking for it?

TITLES WE DIDN'T GIVE THIS BOOK

> Everything You Ever Wanted to Know About Incontinence: Or What to Do with A Wet Cat
> The Sphincter Factor
> Free to Pee (with apologies to Marlo Thomas)
> Don't Let the Rain Come Down
> Out of the Water Closet
> The Drain Game
> Leaking Secrets
> Puddles in the Parlor

SOME ALSO RANS

> Coping with Incontinence from A to P
> Making Waves
> The Book of Floods

ENOUGH?

Ye Olde Tyme Piddler's Manual
The Growth of Minisewage Disposal Devices in the Twentieth
Century

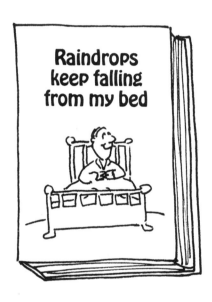

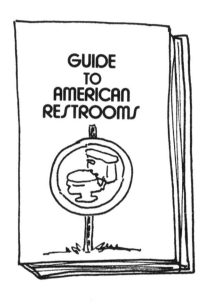

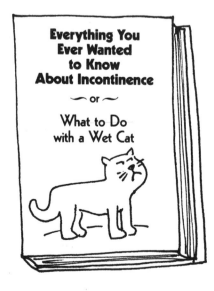

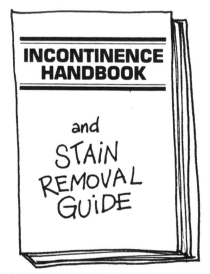

But you needn't take my word that there is humor in incontinence. Listen to others who are affected by it.

MARY JANE: I ask my group what's the worst thing that can happen? Well they bring up all the terrible things that can happen, and I always say I've got a better one than that. And I do have a worse story. Mostly because they are newly incontinent and I have more stories to pull from. And you start realizing that after a while you can look back and laugh. You realized that some of your best friends come out of terrible accidents that happen.

Once I was in the car with a boyfriend and had an accident. I didn't say anything because we were in the middle of nowhere and I was getting almost teary-eyed because there were four more hours of riding. And he said, do you want me to pull into a motel? A person could immediately think, aha, he brought me out here for ulterior motives. But I immediately knew he hadn't. You know, he knew I had had an accident, I wasn't talking about it; he wasn't either.

So we went to this motel where you had to —like people— register by the hour. I went to change my clothes. While I was in there changing my clothes the place was raided. I mean there was this couple down about two doors from us in this building who got raided. I thought when they raided a place they went to every room. My life passed before my eyes. At home I was the saint, the angel; everybody in town thought I was the perfect kid. That's one thing about cripples; they're so good. You know, I saw images of Mary Jane caught in motel raid as headlines in the local paper.

Nobody would have believed that it was because of incontinence . . . and I wouldn't have told them either.

NAN: I think humor has been a tremendous thing in our family. I think everybody has to learn to laugh at themselves and their situation. I remember when I first came home from the hospital and Michael had to stay. I wanted to nurse my baby and they sent me home with an electric breast pump. Joe had me wrap it up in a blanket. Through my tears, I have a picture of me with the electric breast pump wrapped up like a baby sitting in the wheelchair. Believe it or not, it happened to me with my second baby too.

I feel that if I can give that gift to my kids, the gift of being able to find the humor in a situation . . . they will be able to cope.

Nan found out recently how well she had succeeded in giving their child this gift. Michael, a sixth-grader, had gone on his first class trip since his artificial sphincter implantation. Nan waited the day out, worrying over all

73

the things that could go wrong. It was obvious from Michael's face when he came running through the door that something had.

The class had stopped at McDonald's and Michael didn't know what to do. He was surrounded, he told his concerned mother, by a contest poster that proclaimed, "Void Where Prohibited by Law."

MARY JANE: Once I went to a job interview that I was really sure I wasn't going to get. You know, they were looking for a person that

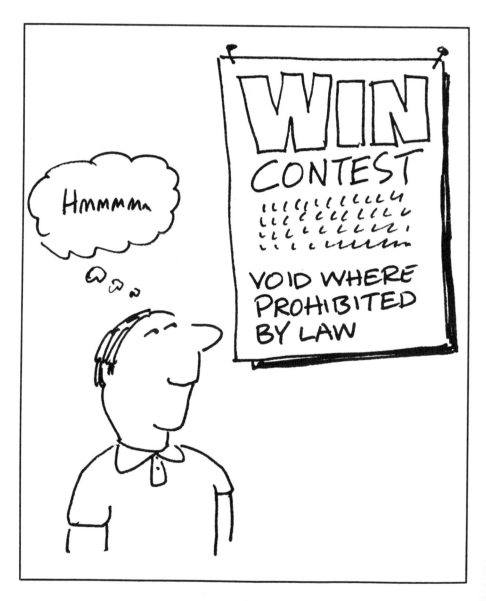

was more experienced than I was. But one of my friends thought I could get it. Anyway, I went to this interview and I was sitting out there, and I kept waiting and waiting. And suddenly, because I was so nervous, I had an accident. I just got up and left. The secretary probably thought I was going for water or something. But I just left.

When I got home the guy who had kept me waiting was on the phone. He thought that I must really be somebody, that I had such intensity that I wasn't going to put up with waiting, even though jobs were hard to get. Sight unseen, he offered me the job.

When a person becomes incontinent he unexpectedly joins the ranks of the differently abled. Following is one man's story about living in the world of the differently abled and how he used humor so effectively as a coping mechanism that he became a comedian and actor.

MAKING OF A COMEDIAN: THE HENRY HOLDEN STORY

During the Vietnam War, all my friends wanted to buy my draft card. You see, I was not going to have to serve my country—I have a physical handicap; I walk with the aid of a leg brace and crutches.

As a child, I never realized that I was handicapped. Crutches were just a tool to help me walk. I didn't see any reason to make a big deal out of it. I never really accepted them—I had no choice in the matter. It was just a natural extension of my being. I had to learn to do everything everyone else did. My crutches were not in my way. In fact, they helped me.

I'll never forget the first time I heard, "He's crippled!"

What a nasty word, *crippled*. I never saw myself as crippled. I thought to myself, did my mind not function? I began to use my mental ability to deal with my physical handicap and I set forth on my own personal philosophy. What the mind can conceive, the man can achieve.

During my first few years in school, I was segregated. I was put into a special class with other handicapped children. According to *Webster's Dictionary, special* means "exceptional," "distinct." But in school it meant "different," with a definite negative connotation.

I was really out of touch with the rest of society. My parents, who certainly meant well, sheltered me from the outside world. In the special class, I was only exposed to others much like me. Outside of school, I noticed that most people were not handicapped—they did not need to use crutches.

Children from the neighborhood would occasionally shout out things to me. "Hey you, cripple!" "Look at Henry, the gimp!" These were, and still are, horrifying words for me to hear. It was then that I said to my parents that I wanted to attend regular school. I wanted to join the others in the mainstream of society. I didn't want to be "special." I wanted to be like everyone else. I wanted to try and compete on an equal level. I decided that I could prove that my crutches would not stand in my way.

The first thing I did was work on mobility. I had to learn to use crutches to the fullest. I taught myself the various techniques of walking with my crutches. I learned how to walk long distances without tiring. I learned how to walk at a faster pace and how to climb stairs. Soon I was moving faster. I couldn't run—but I could move much faster than anyone had thought. Maybe I had something to prove! Unfortunately, there were no role models for me to follow. I had never heard of a famous person with a disability. Maybe I would be the one to influence others with disabilities who were younger than I.

Now, of course, as an adult, I am aware of the many great people throughout history who have contributed to society despite their disabilities. I was never taught about them while in school. I think all students would benefit from learning about the many handicapped personages in history. It is a great feeling to have someone to look up to, to emulate.

While in school, I never asked for special treatment. I didn't expect it, and I didn't want it. I taught myself to deal with the negative comments of the others. I noticed that the more I participated with them, the more respect I got. The saying that respect is earned, not given, is very true.

One thing that was of invaluable help to me was humor. If I could laugh off a negative comment, I would be better off. I let many things roll off my shoulder; didn't take them personally. I thought to myself that their negative attitudes and comments were just mirrors to their own stupidity and immaturity.

As a youngster, I wanted to play sports just like everyone else. Not only could I not run, but I was definitely slower than anyone on the team. So I learned to be a pitcher. If I could be a good pitcher, the fact that I couldn't run would be tolerated. I practiced throwing underhanded with a softball, and overhand with a hard ball. I taught myself how to throw a curve ball similar to the one they throw in the major leagues. I now was able to strike out the opposing batters. In my senior year in high school I was the starting pitcher for our school softball team.

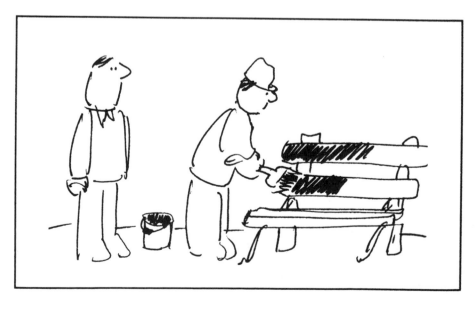

I was the first person with a disability to play on a team at my school, and probably the first in the whole state. Those who assumed that I could not pitch were now strikeout victims. What looks on their faces!

At college I joined the drama department. I was the first disabled person to do so. When my teachers asked me what my goals were, I had a quick response. I wanted to be an actor. One of the instructors pointed out that there had never been a handicapped actor of any reknown. Of course I knew this. But why not? It was time for change. In class I was told that my sense of humor could be used to my advantage. I always used humor to deal with other people's uncomfortableness in dealing with me. Why not turn being funny into a career?

Sure, there are still some people who are uncomfortable when they see my crutches. Merely looking at my crutches startles some. How unfortunate for them! That is their handicap, not mine.

I guess these people think that I should stay home and not be seen. I am trying my best to prove these people wrong. I am not trying to win any awards for courage.

I tell audiences, "Do not applaud just because of my crutches. Don't make a fuss over me. Just treat me like you would any other performer who finds walking a challenge."

My comedy act has been reviewed by several critics. They have called it "original," "provocative," and "inventive." Despite these favorable notices, and my appearance on "Real People," many nightclub owners are hesitant to book me. I've been told by a senior officer at the William Morris Agency [the entertainment industry's largest booking office] that even though he liked the act, it might be offensive to some people.

Why? I don't use any foul language; there are no vile gestures. I guess that the crutches at my side constitute an offense to some people. Not only is this not fair; but it is absolutely without reason or merit.

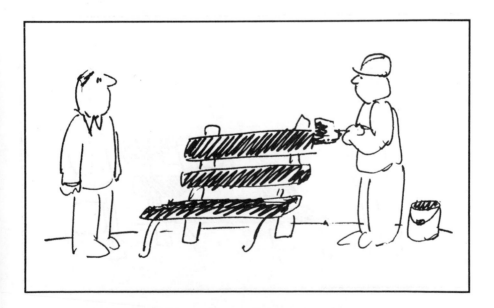

We must influence the youth of this country. Anything should be possible. We must push to have the disabled more visible in the media. The images put forth by these performers would serve to be role models for our nation's youth. There is no way to measure the benefit to a young handicapped child who can identify with someone in the limelight.

Important as this goal is, I never fail to see the lighter side. Some people are uptight about discussing handicap awareness. There is nothing wrong with poking fun at oneself and disabilities:

"New York City recently spent several million dollars installing buses with entrances that kneel down for the handicapped. But I think they have gone too far. Yesterday, I tried boarding one of those modern buses; it knelt down and kissed my ring."

"Did you know that disabled people like me have made their mark throughout history? That's right. In 1450 B.C. King Jerry of Malaysia sang, 'You'll Never Walk Alone' to Siamese twins!"

Up until now I have been using the word *handicapped* or *disabled*. These words are not as bad as *invalid, crippled,* and *maimed,* which are not accurate and should never be used. A new phrase has begun to come into acceptance —*differently abled*. While *handicapped* and *disabled* are often used and are not nearly as offensive as some others, it is my belief that *differently abled* should be given a chance. It connotes a much more positive attitude, and is more accurate.

Day-to-day life can be very challenging, but more so for the differently abled. In today's world we all need patience, but the differently abled also need a good amount of fortitude. They must deal with both physical barriers and attitudinal barriers.

No one can accurately describe what it feels like to have people you have never met form an opinion about you even before you have had a chance to

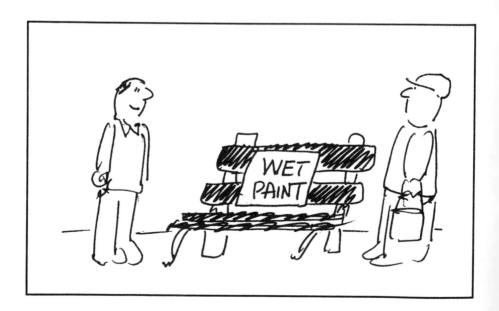

converse. They see my crutches, and I am immediately prejudged. Almost 100 percent of the time it is a negative opinion.

It is very hard to change society's ideas about the differently abled when there are so many roadblocks. We are a multimedia society, and what is seen on television and in the movies molds our perceptions. I feel that it is very important for the differently abled to be more visible in the mainstream of our society.

I have suggested to many of the corporate giants of America that perhaps I could be shown standing in line in a commercial. Or for that matter, any actor or actress, providing that he or she would be in a wheelchair or standing with crutches. Their reply? "Sorry, we can't do that. The public might think that we were playing on their sympathy."

I responded with the suggestion that once in every ten commercials they should hire a differently abled actor. Again, no. Then, perhaps when the camera was focusing in on a table with a happy family, there could be a pair of crutches leaning on the side of the table.

No. The corporate advertisers of America are unwilling to show differently abled people in any manner on their commercials. How hypocritical of them. They will sponsor telethons, they will accept our dollars, but they won't accept us. I know I could do a good commercial for them. Picture this: a thirty-second spot; the camera zooms in on me:

"I can't get along without my crutches. In fact, at tax time, I declare them as a legitimate deduction. These are my American Express crutches— I don't leave home without them!"

If we would come out of our closets, and let the world see that there is nothing wrong with us, it would prove beneficial to everyone. We may be different, but that does not mean anything negative.

There are stigmas connected with the different physical characteristics of

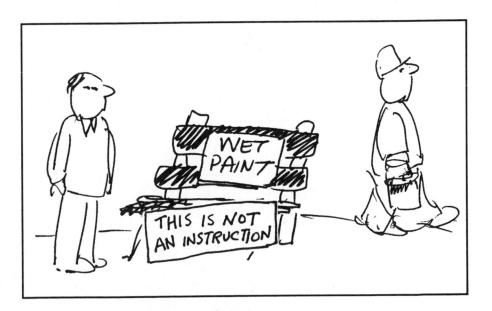

the differently abled. These should not be. Anyone is capable of making a great contribution to society. So many great minds go to waste because of their fear of dealing with society's negative attitudes. I have a lecture titled "Attitudes Are the Real Disability." And how true that statement is.

But the attitudes are on both sides. The differently abled must improve their attitudes too. We should get out of the house, be more visible, and fight the negative attitudes. Prove them all wrong. There is absolutely no reason to be embarrassed by our physical condition.

Both sides need to do much. Together we can change things. We must work together, and I suggest that a little humor will go a long way. We must learn to laugh at ourselves, to see things from a humorous perspective, to learn to accept and appreciate everyone.

"I met a deaf guy who taught himself to talk at age seventy. I asked him why it had taken him so many years to learn. He said that he was lazy and relied on sign language. So why give it up? 'Arthritis,' he replied!"

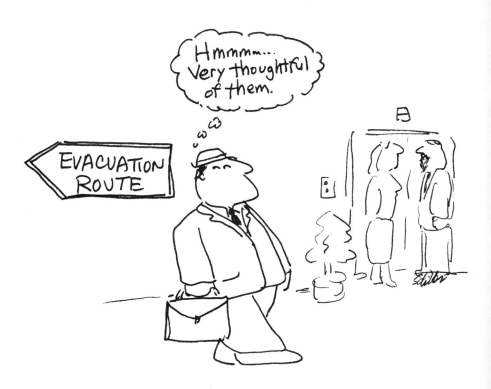

8

Products and Devices for Managing Incontinence

Jane Alvaro
William A. Gartley

INTRODUCTION

This chapter will examine products and procedures that may help you to cope with incontinence. No single method is recommended as the best for any individual. Many devices work well for some persons and not others. If, after trying several devices, you have not found an acceptable product, stop and try to analyze what problems you are having. When you are incontinent, often there are no simple solutions. The following pages contain information that we hope will show you how to manage (not necessarily cure) the incontinence you are experiencing so that the inconvenience and discomfort are lessened. All too often incontinent individuals suffer unnecessarily.

This chapter will define many types of incontinence products that may be useful in helping you, your loved ones, or those for whom you care, live more productive and fuller lives. The products will be described in generic terms rather than by brand to give you a general idea of what types of devices are available. An appendix of product information by manufacturer is included in this book to aid you in finding the products you want to investigate. Please remember that new and improved products are being marketed constantly and many may be comparable to, or better than, the devices described here.

There probably is no perfect product, so begin by choosing the most important features first. Then, as you try products with those features, you can go through the list again, selecting additional features for your needs.

Many people find that one product alone is not completely suitable for all situations. Therefore, we have taken the liberty of categorizing them for different daily activities. As an example, a bulky, highly absorbent product may be very good for nighttime use or for use around the home. For work, or social events, an inconspicuous pad and pant system may be more appropriate. For long confinement periods or long periods of vibration (i.e., traveling for more than two hours on an airplane), an external collection device may be the appropriate coping mechanism.

CHECKLIST OF THINGS TO LOOK FOR

- Absorbency—How long will the product protect you? Will it absorb all the urine you produce without requiring frequent change?
- Bulk—Can the product be seen under normal clothing?
- Disposability—Many products are disposable; some are flushable. Are these important qualities to you?
- Moisture barrier—Many products have a plastic moisture seal. Is it effective in a prone or standing position?
- Noise level—Does the product make noise
  before use?
  during use?
  after use?
- Comfort—Is the product comfortable
  before use?
  after use?
- Changeability—Is the product easy to put on or change? This may be important to people who have arthritis or who have experienced a loss of motor skills.
- Compact—Are extra products easy to carry?
- Availability—Can you get products when you need them?
- Special fitting—Is it required?
- Easy use—How does the product open, close, attach, etc.?
- Special deodorants—Are they required or available?
- Movement—Can the product shift or move when you walk or sit?
- Safety—What causes the product to fail? (For example, some absorbent products seal themselves after contact with a small amount of moisture. Once sealed, they repel moisture.)
- Health—Can long-term use cause skin irritation or other problems?
- Cost—Is the product expensive?
- Is the product discreetly packaged, or available through the mail?

This list is intended to be a guideline. Other features may be important to you that are not listed. Why not stop for a moment and make your own list? Or add to the above list?

ABSORBENT PRODUCTS

Pad and Pants Systems

Pad and pants systems are designed for both men and women to wear under normal clothing. They come in many shapes and sizes and have varying degrees of absorbency. Generally speaking, the system includes an absorbent pad, with moistureproof backing, held next to the body by some type of underpants. Depending on the type of underpants, some people prefer to wear their normal underwear over these systems. Generally, the pads are not too bulky so that spare pads can be carried easily. After use, the pads should be changed relatively soon, disposed of, and a new pad put in place. The pants are generally not changed when the pad is changed.

Pad and Pant systems

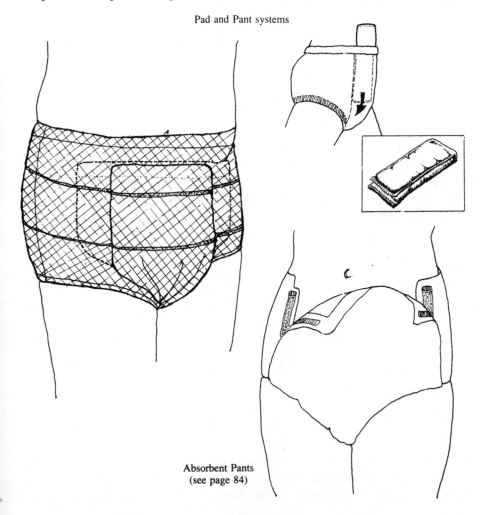

Absorbent Pants
(see page 84)

Certain design features should be kept in mind when looking for pad and pants systems. The pants are sized and manufactured to fit the "average" adult. You may have to experiment to obtain a good fit. Many different types of material are used to absorb urine. Each manufacturer offers specific reasons why its product is the best, but real differences do exist and products must be tried before judged acceptable or not for any individual. Some products have plastic moisture barriers; others do not. Most of these products are designed for collecting urine in a standing or sitting position. Design features for prone and nonambulatory positions should be carefully considered to ensure effective protection.

Absorbent Pants

Absorbent pants are also for the incontinent individual (male or female) who wants to go about normal life activities. Absorbent pants tend to be somewhat bulkier than the pad-pants systems, but many would be acceptable under loose-fitting street wear. Because of their greater bulk, the absorbent pants generally can accommodate greater amounts of urine than the pad and pants systems.

Two features distinguish absorbent pants. Most pants have a built-in moisture barrier (which may cause some rustling noise) and a wide variety of closure devices. It appears that many of the absorbent pants would be simple to change for an arthritic individual or an individual with some loss of motor skills. Closure devices include buttons, velcro strips, adhesive pads, etc. Many of the products offer either front-closing or side-closing products, which may affect ease of use. Again, most of these products come in small, medium, and large, and you may need to experiment to find the size that accommodates your figure.

Absorbent pants can be used by both men and women. Because they are usually completely lined with absorbent material, they can be used sitting, standing, or in a prone position. Since they are somewhat bulkier than most pad and pants systems, it may be more difficult to carry extra supplies to work or social events. Moreover, to date, no absorbent pants are flushable, and that fact makes discreet disposal a consideration.

Adult Undergarments

These are the bulkiest of the garments that can be worn to manage incontinence. Some people will use this type of protection at home or at night and use either a pad and pants system or absorbent pants when out and about. Adult undergarments (known also as adult diapers) are available in both disposable and reusable forms. Some of the disposable products in-

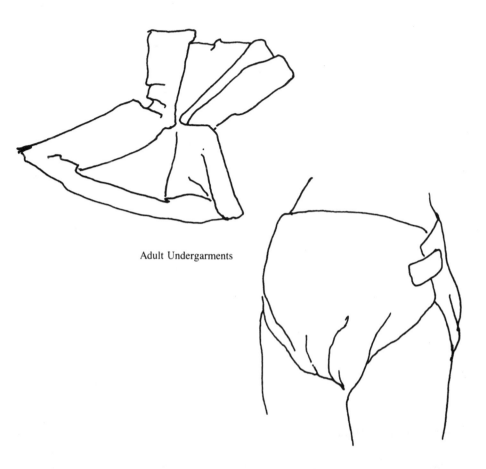

Adult Undergarments

corporate a plastic moisture barrier. Many of these products use velcro and adhesive closure devices, thereby reducing the sizing problem identified with other products. To date, none of these products is flushable, so disposal is a potential problem in a public setting. The products can also be somewhat bulky, so it may be inconvenient to carry a large supply of them.

Drip Collectors for Males

Drip collectors for males are cuplike pouchlike devices that will collect small amounts of urine. Generally, they enclose the penis or the penis and scrotum and are held in place either by means of a belt or by being pinned to the underwear of the individual. The drip collector is useful for work or social settings since it cannot be seen when worn correctly. The interior of the pouch is lined with absorbent material and the exterior of the pouch is a plastic moisture barrier. These small pads can be carried conveniently.

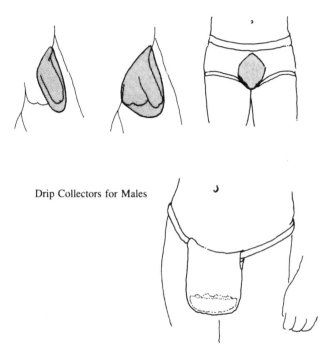

Drip Collectors for Males

They may be an appropriate solution for men who experience only a small amount of urine leakage.

Bed Protection Devices

Some people with urinary incontinence may need protection only at night or may need extra protection at night. Many manufacturers produce a pad

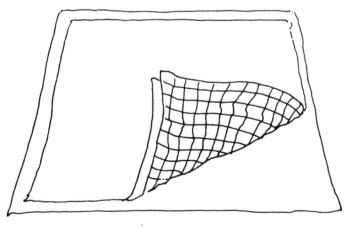

Bed Protection Devices

that can be placed on the bed at hip level to collect urine released while in bed. Most of the disposable bed protection pads have a moisture barrier on the bottom. The pads come in a variety of sizes and absorbency levels. Some may be less expensive than the fitted incontinence devices mentioned previously.

INTERNAL COLLECTION DEVICES

Internal collection devices are for both men and women. These devices, called catheters, are designed for long-term insertion (the Foley catheter) and also for use by individuals at periodic intervals (intermittent catheterization). Devices of this type should be used only under the direction of a physician.

Foley Catheter

Used for long-term catheterization, a Foley catheter is a tube with an inflatable cuff at one end. Deflated, it is inserted into the urethra (the opening of the bladder). The same device is used for both males and females and usually is painless when inserted properly. The deflated cuff is inserted into the bladder past the sphincter muscle. This muscle holds the urine in the bladder and must be released to urinate. Once in position, the cuff is inflated with a small bulb. The inflation causes a ridge or doughnut shape to appear around the tube, thus holding the catheter inside the bladder. The external portion of the catheter is attached to a collection tube that drains into either a leg bag or another collection device. This combination is suitable for work or social events since the leg bag can be concealed. Internal devices require

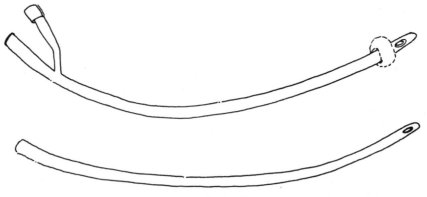

Internal Collection Devices
A. Foley catheter   B. One of a variety of intermittent catheters

87

cleaning of the equipment and frequent emptying of the leg bag, and may increase the risk of a urinary tract infection. Again, this device should be used only under the direction of a physician.

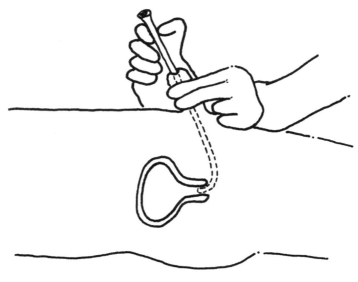

Male being catheterized

Intermittent Catheterization

Intermittent catheterization may be appropriate for patients who have the ability and dexterity to insert a catheter into their own urethra at periodic intervals. Many physicians suggest this be done every three to four hours. One advantage of this method of dealing with incontinence is that the bladder

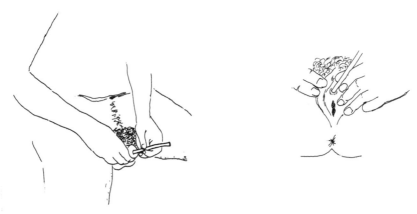

Self-catheterization

can be completely emptied, and residual urine does not collect as a breeding ground for infection. Only certain types of bladder conditions lend themselves to this type of remedy for incontinence. A thorough medical evaluation of the reasons for your incontinence should be done before intermittent catheterization is attempted.

EXTERNAL COLLECTION DEVICES

External collection devices, like the internal ones, require a drainage tube and collection bag. They work in a fashion similar to that of the catheters, except that they surround the penis in the male and are attached to the genital area in females. They are effective when properly placed; however, these devices have been known to loosen at inappropriate times.

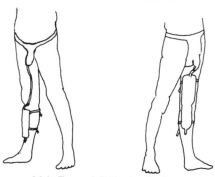

Male External Collection Devices

Male External Collection Devices

The male external collection device is usually a rubber condomlike device that drains into a collection tube. It is held in place by a belt, leg bands, and adhesives. Some men find them quite effective; others have difficulty keeping them in place. Another complication is skin breakdown, caused by too much pressure and often aggravated by constant contact with urine. Like the catheters described previously, the external collection device must be cleaned and the leg bag emptied often.

Female Collection Devices

The woman who is incontinent has fewer choices regarding the type of external collection device that she can use. As one would expect, the greatest obstacle in developing a female external collection device is where and how to attach it.

SURGICAL REMEDIES

There are surgical techniques that may improve the ability to control bladder functions. The best way to determine if you are a potential candidate for the surgery is to discuss it thoroughly with your physician. Since there are differences of opinion about many medical problems, you should be thoroughly informed before making a decision. Seeking a second opinion is often a good idea before undergoing elective surgery.

Artificial Sphincters

Artificial sphincters can be implanted surgically in both male and females. They are doughnut-shaped cuffs that surround the urethra. When operating in a normal position, they fill with fluid and exert an inward pressure on

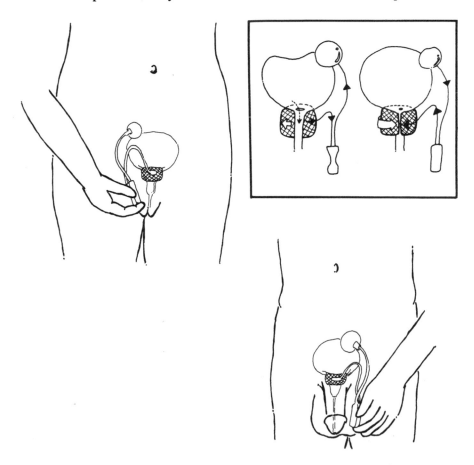

Artificial Sphincters

the urethra. This inward pressure squeezes the urethra closed in a manner similar to a real sphincter muscle. When the individual realizes the urge to urinate, there is time to find a restroom and release the pressure on the urethra by pressing a small bulb (concealed in the scrotum in males and the labia minora in females). This action drains the fluid from the cuff into a self-contained reservoir, allowing the bladder to drain. After a few minutes, the cuff automatically fills with fluid again, closing the urethra. Artificial sphincters have had a high success rate for appropriate bladder problems. They are currently implanted only on carefully screened patients. Please consult with your physician to determine if you are a potential candidate.

Electrical Implants

Manufacturers have experimented with a variety of electrical implants, in which either the sphincter or the bladder walls have been implanted with battery-operated electrodes. Although this may work effectively in theory, practical results have not been satisfactory. As of this writing, we are not aware of electrical implants that are widely recommended. Consult with your physician periodically for news about this area of research.

MUSCLE CONDITIONERS

Certain individuals have a type of incontinence related to weak muscle tone. This is often true for women who have had many childbirths. These women experience what is called stress incontinence . . . the unexpected loss of urine when coughing, laughing, or sneezing. Many of these individuals may respond to muscle-conditioning exercises.

Kegel Exercise

The Kegel exercise is one that you can practice in the privacy of your home. It works by exercising the sphincter muscles around the urethra to build more stamina and endurance in the muscles. The exercise consists of starting and stopping urination several times during the course of normal voiding. The Kegel exercise works well for people in establishing more control. You might want to ask your physician or nurse about using these exercises to help your condition.

Electrical Muscle Conditioners

Electrical muscle conditioners can also be used to strengthen sphincter muscles. These work by creating a low-grade electrical current that causes the muscle to contract. Then the muscle is given a brief rest period before the next electrical stimulus. This process is repeated several times in a given exercise period. Electrical muscle conditioners are, at present, somewhat new to the market.

OTHER DEVICES

Many other devices have been tried over time, some successfully, many not. One device for men that has been used is the penile clamp, which puts pressure on the penis to prevent leakage. Another device, this one for women, is the pessary, a hard rubber doughnut-shaped device that is inserted into the vagina to put pressure on the urethra. When one looks at the history of what has been attempted over the ages to help those with urinary incontinence, it is apparent that managing incontinence has indeed been a challenge.

This chapter was designed to give you a generic overview of what is available to the consumer as of this printing. Since human beings come in all shapes and sizes, and each individual's incontinence is in all likelihood unique, we urge you to experiment. One product may be totally unsuccessful. However, the next one you try may be the right management device for you. There is one way to find out: become determined to manage your incontinence and explore where this determination leads you.

At the end of this book you will find an appendix containing product advertisements. We urge you to read this carefully and write to the manufacturers for more information about their products.

9

Medical Help for Incontinence
William Kaplan, M.D.

The lower urinary tract includes the bladder and urethra. The bladder is designed to hold various amounts of urine for variable periods of time, emptying when full. The urethra is the tube that carries the urine to the outside. The bladder and urethra are similar to a funnel. At the point where the funnel narrows to the spout are two muscles. One is smooth and works involuntarily (without our knowing about it), the other is striated (striped) and works voluntarily (we make it work). When the bladder, or urethra, or muscles work improperly, incontinence occurs.

Additionally, blood vessels and nerves are connected to all these structures in order for them to work properly. The nerves are like telephone wires transmitting messages to and from the brain. All lines go through the main nerve of the body, the spinal cord. Damage to these nerves can occur through injury, disease, or problems at birth. This damage can cause alterations in the way the bladder will fill and empty and in the way the two muscles at the bottom of the bladder will function.

All therapy for incontinence must deal with the bladder or the two sphincter muscles. Your doctor will try to determine if the problem lies in the structure of the bladder and/or sphincter, or whether nerve damage is the cause of the problem. In many cases, however, damage has occurred both to the nerves and to the bladder, and after time it may not be possible to identify which is actually causing the incontinence. It is important to determine the source of the problem, but in practice it is equally important to treat the end result, the incontinence.

The therapy for incontinence is either medical or surgical. Medical therapy is based on the use of exercises or biofeedback, appliances, or drugs. Surgical therapy involves the use of surgery on the bladder or bladder neck, or diversionary surgery, or the implantation of artificial devices.

It is important for your doctor to obtain a complete history and physical examination. Specific radiographic studies may be necessary, such as kidney and bladder X-rays, particularly a bladder X-ray that includes a voiding study. *Urodynamic* assessment may be required. (Urodynamics are studies to determine the function of the bladder and the sphincter muscles.) *Cystoscopy* (the direct observation of the bladder) may be required. Your other health problems should be corrected as well as possible before correction of the incontinence. For example, an individual with a urinary-tract infection and diabetes mellitus will often have an irritable bladder and incontinence. Treatment of the infection and adequate control of the diabetes may be all that are required to treat incontinence.

Your overall general health will often determine your doctor's choice of therapy. Patients with multiple sclerosis will often have perfect urinary control when in remission, only to have severe incontinence with each attack. If the incontinence is only intermittent and not terribly disabling during the exacerbation, your doctor would not resort to radical surgical procedures. On the other hand, a patient who is incontinent because of previous surgery (such as transurethral resection of the prostate) or a stable but disabling neurological condition (e.g., spina bifida) will not have major changes in his or her degree of incontinence and can be treated with this in mind.

People have several basic types of incontinence, and each type requires its own therapy:

1. Patients who have neurologic abnormalities; for example, MS, cerebral palsy, spinal-cord injury, spina bifida.
2. Patients who are neurologically normal; for example, postoperative prostate surgery incontinence or postoperative bladder-neck surgery.
3. Patients who are neurologically normal but anatomically abnormal; for example, pelvic-floor weakness following childbirth, obesity (stress incontinence), or patients with exstrophy-episapadias.
4. Patients who are neurologically and anatomically normal; for example, female urethral syndrome, childhood enuresis (nighttime wetting), or children with voiding abnormalities (daytime and/or nighttime wetting).

Not all abnormalities are included in this brief list, and the treatments that follow may not be specifically matched to each problem. Each individual has different needs and goals, as well as physical and mental capabilities. What follows here is a general review of accepted therapy for incontinence. The specifics, particularly for the different surgical procedures, should be carefully discussed with your doctor.

EXTERNAL DEVICES

Included under this category would be diapers, clothing inserts, condom catheters, external clamps (Cunningham clamp), and internal devices (pessaries).

The condom catheters and Cunningham clamp require special care. The Cunningham clamp and the condom catheter are placed around the penis, and therefore great care is needed to be certain that blood flow to the penis is not compromised. The condoms and clamp should be removed at night to air out the skin to prevent ulcer formation. For many individuals with minimal incontinence or occasional incontinence, clothing devices, inserts, etc., may be the best choice. Individuals who have gained good urinary control may wish to wear these devices as merely insurance or when they are under stress. These devices can be used as an adjunct to any of the forthcoming therapies.

CLEAN INTERMITTENT CATHETERIZATION

Except for female stress incontinence and postsurgical incontinence (particularly prostate surgery), the standard that other types of treatment are measured against is clean intermittent catheterization (CIC). CIC may be effective in the above exceptions; however, surgery is usually the treatment for female stress incontinence and an artificial sphincter is the usual treatment for postsurgical incontinence.

CIC was introduced three decades ago as the initial therapy for patients with spinal-cord injury. Over the years, numerous reports have documented that CIC reduces the incidence of *pyelonephritis* (kidney infection), *hydroureteronephrosis* (kidney and ureter swelling), *reflux* (urine backing up into the kidneys from the bladder), and kidney and/or bladder stones. CIC alone has significantly reduced the need for urinary diversion in patients with incontinence.

The procedure is simple. The hands and an appropriately sized catheter are washed with soap and water. The urethral opening (*meatus*) is washed, and the catheter is inserted into the bladder. All the urine is drained, and the catheter is washed again and stored. This process is repeated every three to four hours during the daytime and occasionally as needed once in the middle of the night. In our experience, there is no child too young, male or female, for this procedure. If manual dexterity is present, no individual is too old for the procedure. Children can generally be trained to perform self-catheterization between the ages of four and six. In our myelomeningocele population, with the addition of pharmacotherapy in 80 percent of the patients, 85 percent of the children are dry for three to four hours with this program.

Intermittent catheterization is less effective or not desirable when there is total sphincter incompetence (that is, the sphincter muscle below the bladder does not function or has been traumatically or surgically injured), or urethral stricture (narrowing), or disease, or severe uninhibited bladder contractions (bladder contracts with little control or forewarning) that are not controlled with medication.

SURGICAL THERAPY

The most common category of incontinence that is probably best managed surgically is female stress incontinence. This most often arises from childbirth, age, or obesity or any combination thereof. Relaxation of the pelvic floor (the muscles that support the bladder, urethra, uterus, and vagina) is also noted more frequently with serious joggers. The symptoms of stress incontinence can be quite severe and disabling. The incontinence occurs with a sudden change in position, or with laughter, coughing, or lifting of objects.

Diagnosis is based on an accurate history, physical examination, and voiding X-ray studies. Commonly the diagnosis is made by inserting a catheter into the urethra and leaving behind a beaded chain within the bladder and urethra to evaluate various angles of the urethra relative to the bladder (*chain cystogram*). A *cystometrogram* (pressure study) of the bladder should be done to be certain that one does not have uninhibited bladder contractions. A Marshall test is also helpful in the diagnosis. This requires the physician to place fingers on either side of the urethra and ask the patient to strain or cough. If leakage is prevented when the fingers are elevated, surgical success is likely.

Sophisticated examinations, X-rays, and pressure studies have recognized two types of abnormal anatomy that cause stress incontinence: Type I and Type II. Simply, Type I is best managed with a vaginal operation to tighten the pelvic musculature, and Type II will require surgery just above the pubic area. (The incision will be just above the hard pelvic bone in the front.) The surgery for the Type II problem requires hitching the bladder and urethra into a higher position.

High cure rates for females with stress incontinence rely on accurate diagnosis with X-rays and pressure studies (*urodynamics*) before the choice of surgical approach. For skilled surgeons, these repairs can be very successful, and though drugs and intermittent catheterization may be helpful as an adjunct to treatment, the best course of therapy for this problem is generally surgical.

Surgery may also be most helpful when there is total sphincteric incompetence from trauma, or prostate surgery, or neurologic injury.

ARTIFICIAL URINARY SPHINCTER

Individuals with total sphincteric incompetence are probably best managed with the artificial urinary sphincter. The new-generation semiautomatic artificial urinary sphincter (800 series) from the American Medical Systems has been manufactured with great care and appears to be reliable. Your doctor may decide to insert an artificial sphincter if the following criteria are met:

1. The bladder does not have uninhibited contractions or is controlled by medication.
2. The patient can empty the bladder to completion or perform CIC.
3. Reflux (urine backing up to the kidneys) is not present.
4. The patient has good manual dexterity to operate the sphincter.
5. There has been a complete neurourologic workup.
6. All conservative measures, such as CIC and aggressive drug therapy, have failed.

The artificial urinary sphincter has been used more frequently in adults than in children. However, several institutions are now able to insert and care for the sphincter in the child. In adult males the sphincter can be placed around the bladder neck, or lower on the urethra. In children and women it *must* be placed around the bladder neck. Five-year success rates approach 90 percent in adults, although within the five years, one or more revisions of the sphincter components may be necessary. There is not yet as much long-term experience with the artificial sphincter in children. Only extensive trials will determine its true rate of success in both adults and children.

The sphincter is easily operated. It always remains closed except when it is manually opened. It remains open for three to seven minutes. The bladder is then emptied (either naturally or with the use of a catheter). It then closes automatically. The greatest problems with the sphincter are malfunction and infection of the device. Malfunction may be remedied by replacing the part that works improperly. However, infection can be severe enough to warrant removal. In either case, the end results could be erosion of the urinary tract. Erosion is the wearing away of the tissue beneath the cuff, that is, the urethra or bladder neck. When this occurs, the cuff will protrude through the bladder neck or urethra. Appropriate cuff and balloon pressure selection can help to minimize erosion, though it can still occur even under the best of conditions. In adult males who have had a previous urethral cuff, a new cuff can be placed around the bladder neck. In children and women with previous bladder-neck cuffs, erosion often eliminates future cuff placement.

In view of the fact that the artificial sphincter is made from silicone and can become infected or fatigued, many surgeons prefer other surgical techniques to placement of the artificial device.

The list of procedures that have been tried is extensive. It is certainly true that the history of the treatment of urinary incontinence is characterized by trial, error, early rejoicing, and late frustration. With nearly all procedures, the goal is to slow down the flow. This can be accomplished by changing the slant or compressing the urethra or lengthening the bladder-neck area. Many surgical procedures have been designed to accomplish this goal, and in selected cases success can be achieved.

DRUG THERAPY

The use of medication in the treatment of urinary incontinence is based on two major approaches. The first is to get the bladder to relax and/or expand to prevent uninhibited bladder contractions. The drugs most often used for this purpose are those that block the discharge signals for the bladder contraction, namely, Pro-Banthine or Ditropan. The second major approach is to cause constriction of the outlet of the bladder. Drugs used for this purpose would be Ephedrine or Ephedrine-like drugs. (Most cold tablets contain these products.)

The two approaches presume that the bladder is able to empty to completion. When the bladder does not contract or empty effectively, this may also cause incontinence. Effective emptying may require other drugs or a catheter (CIC) or surgery. Occasionally the bladder can contract either perfectly or fairly well, but the muscles below the bladder do not relax appropriately and the bladder never fully empties. This is called *vesical sphincter dyssynergia* (discoordination of the bladder muscle with the sphincter muscle). True vesical sphincter dyssynergia occurs in diseases of the nervous system. It can be most difficult to treat successfully. It may require the use of all types of treatment—surgery, medication, and intermittent catheterization.

Finally, in children and in young adults, inappropriate voiding or ineffective voiding can cause incontinence. Normal voiding is a learned response that requires maturity of many body systems. Often in the toilet-learning process, poor habits develop. This can lead to daytime or nighttime wetting, or both. Appropriate toilet habits generally develop between three and six years of age. Wetting beyond this age may be a problem. Again, a thorough history and physical examination, and perhaps X-rays and urodynamics, may be necessary for a proper diagnosis and treatment plan.

In older children and young adults, medication may be effective. However, some individuals may benefit from a retraining process or biofeedback. Through urodynamics, individuals can actually observe their urinary flow and muscular activity and correct for incoordination that may be causing the wetting. The biofeedback training is effective only in selected cases and requires an intact neuromuscular system. An additional variation on biofeedback is available in a few centers. This system is not totally dependent on a completely intact neuromuscular system, but does require good sensation (that is, the patient must be able to feel bladder distention). It involves intermittent electrical stimulation to the bladder via a catheter. Sessions generally last ninety minutes a day, seven days a week, for months. Success with this electrical biofeedback can be achieved, though retreatment is usually required.

Incontinence can be very disabling. Only through an aggressive, creative approach to treatment, with active participation by the patient, family, friends, and professional staff, can success be achieved.

10

Sexuality and Incontinence
Rosemarie B. King, R.N., M.S.

Incontinence can affect a person's sexuality and confidence in various ways:

1. Loss of bladder control can result in feelings of being less masculine or feminine.
2. Fear of urine leakage during intimacy can create anxiety.
3. Concerns about management of urinary appliances during sexual contact can affect confidence.

These concerns often remain unspoken, but there are few incontinence issues which cannot be resolved by a willing couple. Resolution of these problems requires communication between the partners. If it is difficult for you to start a discussion about sex with your partner (it is for most people), it may help to ask him or her to read this section and then to discuss the information that applies.

Men and women are frequently embarrassed to discuss incontinence with their doctor. For many, it's even harder to express sexual concerns. Many doctors and nurses are now trained to deal with this subject. Family practitioners, urologists, psychiatrists (specialists in physical disability), and gerontologists (specialists in care of older persons) frequently encounter sexual questions. Nurses in these fields are also excellent resources. Don't worry about shocking them or thinking that you're the only one with sexual concerns. In reality, almost everyone with loss of bladder control has questions in this area and many health professionals will anticipate your concern. Unfortunately, many professionals worry that they will offend the client, and won't ask about this area of life. But if you raise questions, they usually can help or can refer you to an expert resource.

There are numerous reasons for the hesitancy to be open about sexual matters. Myths and taboos have long existed about sexual practices and body parts. As children, many of us were told "don't touch" if we touched our genitals. When sexual questions were asked of parents or teachers, embarrassment and abrupt responses were likely. How often do children see parents touching or cuddling each other? Children soon get the message that sexuality is not something one talks about.

Myths tend to be passed from generation to generation. These myths can distort our view of sexuality and have the potential to inhibit our sexual pleasure and that of our partner. Examples of some common myths are listed below:

MYTH	CORRECTION
Intimate touch should result in intercourse and orgasm.	Intimate touch can be erotic and pleasurable in and of itself.
Disabled persons are not sexual.	A person with a disability is as sexual as an able-bodied person. Depending on the disability, certain sexual acts may not be possible, but many options for sexual expression are open.
The genitals in a male and female, and the female breasts are the only sexual organs.	Untrue. The largest sexual organ is the skin. Many parts of the body have exquisite sensation; they are capable of pleasurable, erotic sensations. Examples are lips, tongue, ears, neck, breasts of female and male, fingertips, spine, etc.
Older persons aren't interested in sex and don't enjoy it. (This myth and the one about disabled persons reflect our society's emphasis on youth, beauty, and body physique.)	Untrue. Older men and women remain sexual. Some changes occur in sexual response of the body and in energy level, but many older persons continue sexual activity into very old age. Figure 1.

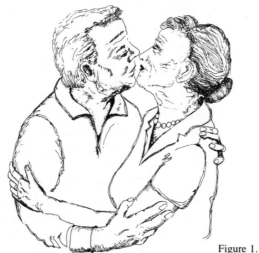

Figure 1.

| Masculinity and femininity depend on the number of people who are sexually attracted to you and the frequency of intercourse. | Not true. Sexuality is the way we express our femaleness and maleness. If we think of it in this way, then masculinity and femininity include: (1) the way we dress and act; (2) our image of ourself; (3) our roles as mothers and fathers, husbands, wives or lovers; and (4) specific acts such as caressing, hugging, kissing, and intercourse. Thus, it is far more than the number of sexual attractions and intercourse. Too much emphasis on performance can actually dilute sexual pleasure. Our society places great emphasis on performance of sexual acts. |

By now you have the idea: these myths can, for some people, end up dictating their sexual relationship. In reality the couple should decide between them what is okay and pleasurable. Much of the joy and pleasure possible with sexual contact can be lost if a couple doesn't communicate. Lovemaking without the sharing of other parts of oneself, and of what is physically pleasurable for each, diminishes the feeling of intimacy and pleasure. Developing the ability to give and to receive feedback concerning intimacy issues is even more important when loss of bladder control exists.

Very early in life we begin to develop an image of ourself as a person who is acceptable and lovable to others by being touched, held, and cuddled. We also get in touch with our bodies and learn about the differences between boys and girls by exploring our bodies and those of playmates. Sexual curiosity is a normal part of growing up; the questioning, and playing doctor or mommy/daddy are routine in a child's life. Sometimes parents are disturbed when children touch themselves, and discourage this activity, not realizing how normal it is.

Depending on the parent's reaction, a child may feel he is doing something wrong and feel guilty. These feelings can be enduring and one can grow up believing it is wrong to touch oneself or another in pleasurable ways.

Another activity that contributes to the child feeling accepted is learning control of elimination activities. Control of bowel and bladder functions is given such importance by parents, especially mothers, that a child believes that control of these functions is quite a feat. They generally feel proud of their accomplishment and may even be proud of the waste that leaves their body. In our society, a child soon learns that adults consider body waste with some degree of disgust. Accomplishing control of elimination is considered "grownup." Parents will say, "What a big girl!" when control is gained. Or they may scold a child who loses control. These experiences are, in part, the basis for feeling undesirable when incontinence exists.

Attitudes and actions of health professionals can also contribute to a negative self-image when chronic illness requires frequent physical examination or hospitalization, or both. If privacy issues are ignored or parts of the body are examined in an undignified manner, the person can begin to think less of himself.

The close proximity of sexual organs to organs of urination can result in misconceptions about body parts and confusion about feeling clean or unclean. Many girls and women don't understand their sexual anatomy, especially where sexual organs are located in relationship to urinary opening. The meatus (urinary opening) is not normally located in the vagina as many women believe. However, the close proximity to the anal opening requires good hygiene to prevent infections. The clitoris is an organ whose only purpose is sexual pleasure. Because it is located a little distance from the vagina, some females and their partners are not fully aware of its presence and purpose as a source of pleasurable sensations and focus only on vaginal stimulation. Understanding these body parts is helpful when considering sexuality issues and incontinence. Male sex organs, unlike those of females, are readily visible and it's obvious that the urinary opening is located in the head of the penis. The visibility of the male organ does allow much comparison of penis size, especially among adolescent boys. It's not unusual for boys to feel inferior if their penis size doesn't compare favorably with that of others in the locker room. A basic fact that is not well understood is that the size of a flaccid penis has nothing to do with getting an erection and the ability to share pleasurable intercourse.

EXPRESSIONS OF INTIMACY

For a number of social reasons, a majority of persons do not grow up with a great deal of comfort about sexual matters. One expert in the field, Sol Gordon, professor of child and family studies at Syracuse University, encourages parents to find a way to initiate a conversation when uncomfortable. Perhaps an indirect method such as referring to a newspaper article can be used. Parents can also refer to books, and that approach may help them to bring up the topic of sexuality. Just as parental communication with children is essential to the child's education, communication between lovers is critical to a satisfactory, loving relationship. The question "How was I" or "How was it" is not exactly the type of communication to which I'm referring. Communication between lovers may be through the spoken word or nonverbally through the eyes, a hug, body posture, or touch. An affectionate, loving touch can express so much feeling and intimacy.

It's helpful to share with a partner where you like to be touched, or perhaps, guide your partner's hand. This is even more important when a device such as a catheter is present, or if one has no sensation or experiences pain in parts of the body. Most experts consider any sexual activity between consenting partners which is acceptable to both to be normal. However, many people in our culture consider only certain activities or positions to be appropriate for them. It's important to check out and to share what each considers acceptable and pleasurable or exciting. Lovers often will compromise; for example, one may be unsure about a sexual activity that the partner desires but will experiment to please the lover. Usually, reluctance to experiment traces to concern over normalcy of the act. Many in our society aren't knowledgeable about the range of possibilities and the variety of needs of much of the population. However, reluctance to participate in certain sexual activities must always be respected.

Close body contact is an excellent way to communicate love and affection. Unclothed lovers, lying together, can create intimate, relaxing, or very stimulating sensations, depending on the mood and the desires of the couple.

When a health problem such as incontinence exists, it's helpful to set the stage for intimate contacts. For most people with the problem, intimate sexual contact is easier when the partner is well known and the opportunity to gauge sensitivity has occurred. This enables one to come up with an approach to explaining incontinence to a partner. There are a number of ways of approaching the subject. In the film *Coming Home*, Jon Voight doesn't explain or discuss incontinence issues with Jane Fonda. He chooses to undress in another room and remove or adjust bladder drainage equipment. Many people prefer to mention to their lover the possibility of dribbling urine or that a device must be removed and reapplied. A woman with a catheter will want to explain that she leaves the tube in place and to guide her partner in adapting techniques a bit. For some, it may be easier to give a book to read with passages marked that relate to a particular problem. In some situations, the partner will need to assist in removing, applying, or adjusting appliances. This can be incorporated into lovemaking, and performed as a part of sex play. Certain couples decide to have an attendant assist with care. This may be done when paralysis or weakness prohibits independent function in dressing and undressing, getting in and out of bed, and manipulating urinary equipment or programs.

If you are fearful of getting involved with others because you think that they would be turned off by your incontinence or devices, or that you could never explain, it can be helpful to talk to a skilled health professional such as a psychologist, or nurse, or social worker. These professionals can often help individuals to feel more at ease in bringing up the subject, and in dealing with potential rejection. You probably will not feel totally comfortable, but will not freeze at the thought of discussing this delicate topic.

MANAGING INCONTINENCE DURING SEXUAL ACTIVITY

Looking and feeling sexual is a main first step in handling incontinence issues during intimacy. For some, it's helpful to set the mood with soft lights, music, and perhaps some wine. Others will feel more sexy in certain outfits or lingerie, or if they smell good. If you can feel good about yourself and are relaxed, you are less likely to be worried about incontinence issues and can approach them in a matter-of-fact way.

Let us look at some of the incontinence concerns that many people experience and outline some approaches to these concerns.

Dribbling a small amount of urine during sexual excitement or intercourse is experienced by many women at various times. If weakness of the pelvic-floor muscles (the ones that run along the genital, lower buttock, and anal area) exists, Kegel's exercises may help. These exercises (described elsewhere in this book) consist of regularly tightening the muscles to strengthen them. In this way leakage of urine is avoided. It also helps to empty the bladder just before sexual contact. Men can apply a condom to contain the small amount of urine they may lose.

Incontinence of large amounts of urine creates feelings of embarrassment for most. Having an understanding partner minimizes the worry about this happening. It is necessary to be prepared; bedclothing can be protected with large towels or underpads; have extra towels and washcloths or large pre-moistened towelettes handy to cleanse self and partner. You may be able to prevent the incontinence with some precautions. Empty your bladder before intercourse and avoid fluids for an hour before activity. If incontinence does occur and concern about transmission of a urinary infection exists, your partner should empty his or her bladder immediately, wash the genital area well, and then drink several glasses of water to wash out any bacteria that may have entered the bladder. Reports of urinary infection transmitted during intercourse are uncommon in the medical literature on incontinence.

What can you say or do should incontinence occur during loving moments? Usually *not* helpful are getting very upset, and expressing frustration and anger. Your partner is likely to feel awkward and embarrassed. You may feel upset inside, but if you remain calm and are matter-of-fact about the incident, or perhaps interject humor (if that is your style), it will help both of you to deal with the situation.

Internal catheters (indwelling Foley) can be left in place during foreplay and intercourse or removed, depending on preference. However, since re-

105

sterilization of indwelling catheters is not generally recommended, removal of a catheter can be expensive if you enjoy intercourse regularly.

A male with an internal catheter inserted through the penis can fold the catheter back on the penis and then apply a condom. The condom can be taped in place and well lubricated with a water-soluble lubricant. A vaseline or oil-based lubricant should not be used as infection could occur. This technique is not without some hazard because tugging or traction on the catheter can result in bleeding and infection. However, liberal lubrication reduces the possibility of trauma. The partner will not experience pain with this technique. The issue of catheters is less complicated for females.

A woman can tape the catheter to the lower abdomen, using care not to tug or put tension on the catheter when taping it. She should also inform her partner to avoid activity that causes pulling on the catheter or friction around the urinary opening. If irritation to the urinary opening is a problem when the women is in the astride or bottom (missionary) position, the couple might experiment with rear entry positions.

The presence of a urostomy is no impediment to sexual activities. Some individuals may wish to cover the urostomy or catheter drainage bag; covers can be made from any fabric.

When an external catheter is worn to contain incontinence, it can be removed before sexual activity; fluids should be avoided for an hour or so before contact. The bladder is then emptied by usual techniques. For some, this will be tapping over the bladder; for others, the crede maneuver. Whichever method is used, time is needed to be sure the bladder is empty.

Individuals who manage bladder emptying with intermittent catheterization can catheterize just before sexual contact. If fluids are limited before that time, it's unlikely that the bladder will fill with much urine.

Some may be concerned that urine will be released from the bladder during orgasm. This doesn't happen as often as one might think because the sphincter muscle tightens during orgasm and ejaculation. However, damage to nerves that control this area will interfere with this action and incontinence could occur.

Additional considerations relate to fears that a partner may have and concerns about positioning when fatigue or weakness is part of the condition causing incontinence. As previously stated, a partner may fear exposure to urinary infection or may believe that the person with incontinence will develop a urinary infection. As long as tugging on the catheter and irritating contact with the urinary opening are avoided, an infection is not likely. However, emptying the bladder after intercourse and drinking lots of fluids are additional precautions.

At first a lover may be hesitant about touching tubes and drainage devices. The hesitancy is sometimes from fear of causing harm and sometimes because of distaste for such equipment. If discomfort exists, it is best to handle the equipment yourself. With time, a comfort level will develop and activity such as removing a catheter can be incorporated into lovemaking.

If contractures of joints or weakness of trunk or extremities exists, various positions can be tried. The male who has difficulty assuming the top position during intercourse may find that side-lying, sitting, standing, or the female astride position is more comfortable. Likewise, females may want to experiment with positions that are less fatiguing and allow more movement or control. A thought to keep in mind is that deep penetration of the penis is not necessary for exciting, pleasurable sensations or orgasm for either party. The entrance of the vagina and the clitoris are very sensitive. The last inch or so of the penis is the most sensitive. If you have trouble thinking of positions, a book such as *The Joy of Sex* by Alex Comfort or other books available at your local bookstore may prove helpful. However, sexual excitement and sexual communication do not require penis-vagina intercourse. Alternative methods, mentioned earlier, can bring sexual satisfaction.

In summary, incontinence is not an impediment to a full, satisfying sexual life. It may present some barriers, but they are barriers that can be overcome with imagination and a few simple techniques. Developing communication skills and an openness to sexuality as a total experience enhances dealing with incontinence-related issues in a sexual relationship.

RECOMMENDED READING

Comfort, Alex. *The Joy of Sex*. New York: Simon & Schuster, 1972.
Laireman, Connie, "Teenagers & Sex: Knowledge Is Power" *Chicago Tribune*, November 22, 1983.

11

Incontinence Is Everyone's Problem

Larry P. Horist

Incontinence is a personal health problem, with indirect, but specific, meaning for those with responsibility or affection for those afflicted. If it were a condition affecting only a minuscule proportion of the population, the public would have little reason to elevate the issue to general awareness. The medical community could justify the appropriateness of relegating its treatment to a few specialists.

This is not the case. Incontinence, in one form or another, affects millions of Americans. Incontinence impacts in very meaningful ways on our overall social, economic, and political structure. It results in lost productivity. It has damaging psychological side effects. The economic impact of the loss of social participation is staggering.

This alone does not make incontinence unique. Many afflictions produce similar results, some with even more dramatic and direct consequences. What is unique is that this condition, which involves some ten to twelve million Americans, receives such little public attention. Like Suzie's pregnancy, Uncle Harry's drinking problem, and the hole in the carpet, it is politely hidden from public view.

More than half of all nursing-home patients suffer from incontinence. A significant percentage of them were admitted for that reason alone. In our "enlightened" society people who could continue to make a contribution to society are institutionalized by loved ones who choose to address the problem of incontinence by avoiding it. Unfortunately, the family is not alone in perpetuating this injustice.

Too often, the medical community ignores the potential of corrective measures in older individuals, choosing instead to view incontinence as a frequent and natural condition of aging—something to be accepted, not diagnosed, treated, and managed. This view is similar to the approach dentists took a generation ago when they treated patients as if the good Lord gave them seventy year bodies fitted with forty year teeth.

This tendency to ignore the problem is manifest in many ways. The media generally refuse to carry ads for incontinence products. It is not considered a suitable subject for general circulation publications or the electronic media. Even semispecialty publications, including those directed to senior citizens, refuse to carry such ads. One publisher said the ads would be "too depressing" for its older readership. They do carry ads for wheelchairs, however—not exactly one of your upbeat products.

Public service advertising—those announcements of public interest which the radio and television stations air free of charge in time slots only an insomniac could appreciate—also avoids incontinence. Stations will provide information on everything from the garden club's auction to AIDS, but nothing on incontinence.

The creative advertising industry, which has produced "virile" smoking ads and "tender" contraceptive ads, seems incapable to date of producing an informative and tasteful ad for various incontinence options. The problem rests with both the advertising agencies and the media's standards boards, which tend to ban such advertisements or censor them until they are so bland as to be useless to the consumer.

This lack of information advertising is more than a denial of a manufacturer's right to market a product. It infringes on the rights of the consumer. These arbitrary restrictions deny those suffering from incontinence much needed information on various product options and qualities. In the media, society deals in detail with sweaty armpits, menstruation, vaginal hygiene, loose "choppers," and birth control. We should therefore be ready for incontinence. It is inconceivable that a "novice" product with such a sizable market should be banned from the general media.

Although we think of the United States as a progressive and an increasingly enlightened society, we are faced with two realities: other nations are in the lead in addressing this issue, and as a society we appear to be regressing. In England, the Disabled Living Foundation has an Association of Continence Advisers. Its role is to promote better understanding of the problem within the medical profession and among the general public. In 1983 the Netherlands began a national public education campaign with a direct message: "Over 500,000 Dutch people are incontinent. Isn't it time we talked about it?" Sweden has a specialty publication boldly titled *Inkontinens*.

Not only is the United States behind many other nations of the world; we may be regressing. In the 1920s the Sears Roebuck catalogue offered "high-grade soft rubber urinal bags." These products, for men and women, were described in detail and included illustrations. There were "day and night styles" featuring "valves arranged to prevent return of urine from lower bag." The male design "holds the entire scrotum." Potential buyers were advised to consult physicians before ordering. The absence of euphemisms in these earlier general-circulation catalogues is striking. The products were boldly advertised for "general incontinence of urine." In the Roaring Twenties a household catalogue used the words *scrotum* and *urine*. Today, general advertising outlets avoid the subject. What has happened? There are many answer to that question.

The American society has come to exalt perfection. It seems natural, therefore, to shun those subjects and persons that suggest human frailty—especially those associated with physical manifestations. People with missing limbs and facial disfigurements, for example, are secondarily victimized by an array of inconsistent public reactions, including obvious avoidance, pitiful patronization, and even unconscionable hostility.

Afflictions and conditions that speak to the quality of our body rather than to its general soundness cause even greater problems. Virility in men, fertility in women, and general mental acuity, for example. Incontinence falls into this category.

Incontinence suggests a lack of control. It involves a body function which only the highest mammal seems psychologically ill equipped to deal with.

We humans live in a world that almost denies bodily functions, and certainly punishes the loss of control over the function. We "clean after each use." Powder. Deodorize. Even among our own gender, we hide in little stalls. Men with "bashful bladders" find it difficult to urinate in the company of other men without "concealing" urinals. Even the audible escaping of gas in a social setting is akin to eating soup with your hands.

This attitude of control at all costs is not without its tragic consequences. Most individuals who suffer a loss of control immediately retreat from the larger world. They become incapacitated as much by their own attitude—nurtured by an intolerant society—as by the physical limitations of incontinence itself. There are instances where patients have chosen death over a colostomy.

Thus, we are dealing with an issue that cannot simply be brought to the fore of public awareness like a proposal to balance the federal budget or a new flavor of ice cream. And public awareness is exactly what the topic of incontinence needs to make long-overdue changes in the attitudes of society. However, the issue must be developed on many fronts at the same time.

The fact that incontinence is not a single problem complicates dealing with this issue at a public level. Incontinence is not a disease, an injury, or an emotional or psychological disability. It is the result, the byproduct, of any one of these. Consequently, doctors often focus their medical attention on the primary problem—cancer, spinal injury, infection, etc.—with only secondary concern for the incontinence itself.

And because incontinence is caused by a wide range of physical and emotional problems, it is also difficult to focus public attention or direct action upon it. Most public education programs are geared to specific diseases. There are highly visible campaigns to fight cancer or multiple sclerosis. There are public campaigns that address the causes of diseases—antismoking efforts, for example. Successful public education efforts seem to center on single diseases or single causes. Incontinence does not fit perfectly into either of those categories. It is, however, an affliction with a wide range of common attributes. To build public awareness successfully, it is those common attributes that must be emphasized. Others can be left to address the wide range of causes.

Another stumbling block in developing public awareness of the consideration for incontinence is that it is perceived to be an affliction without potential resolution. Curing cancer is a noble crusade. People remember how public attention and financial resources helped eradicate smallpox and virtually wipe out polio. A sense of purpose and the promise of success marked those efforts. With incontinence perceived as a permanent, unmanageable condition, the lack of public concern is understandable.

To move incontinence to the fore of public awareness we must first define the scope of the problem in larger social terms. Although an array of statistics is available, this information must be assembled in a format that presents a more complete picture of the social and economic impact of the problem. We need to know more than the number of afflicted, their age, sex, and cause. From the public's standpoint, there are more relevant questions. How many lost workdays result from the condition? What is the impact on insurance rates? How much medicaid and medicare money is used on incontinence? What industries lose dollars? What industries gain dollars? Public attention cannot be directed simply because the condition affects legions of people, and because "isn't that a shame." The public must be made to understand fully the social consequences of incontinence. Then action will follow.

The antitobacco lobby is a good example. This issue became successful only after lobbyists were able to interest the nonsmoking public. For years, the lobby tried to convince smokers to quit (without much success); to convince nonsmokers to take up the cause (without much success); and to get government to regulate the business (without much success). After the antismoking groups shifted their public campaign to the secondary effects on the nonsmoker—people in offices with smokers, the family of a smoker, the fetus of a smoking mother-to-be, and so forth—the national effort went into high gear. They involved the previously uninvolved. And once the issue gained a broader base of support, it became "political," and government began to act. Incontinence, like smoking, has a tremendous effect on all of society, an effect not yet defined or recognized by the nonafflicted victims.

Making statistical information relevant to society in general and broadening the support base are preliminary elements of the public education campaign. Actually getting that information before the public is a challenge in itself. Unlike the earlier tobacco analogy, incontinence does not have a willing partner in the media. Those working on the problem are prevented from molding public opinion by a reluctant media. The first effort must be to convince the media to become part of the education process.

Television offers the greatest opportunity to reach the lives of Americans of all social and economic conditions. Unfortunately, the highly graphic nature of the medium may make it the most difficult with which to deal on the subject of incontinence.

Initially, the best potential television will be public-affairs talk shows and interview spots. These programs are constantly looking for new causes. An issue that has not been fully explored in public is a natural for them. If it is controversial, so much the better.

A fairly new trend in television is on-air science-health news reporters. These specialized reporters tend to break new ground in subjects discussed and illustrated on the airwaves.

Cable television offers a rare opportunity to bring the issue of incontinence into the home. Because of the vast number of stations and their ability to present programming directed at smaller specialty markets, cable is always looking for "lifestyle" programs. There are even special channels devoted to health issues. Perhaps a regularly scheduled program could be devoted specifically to incontinence. Cable television becomes a surprisingly private and personal medium to bring incontinence information into the homes of the afflicted. Religious programs, with their emphasis on overcoming human problems, are another potential outlet for the education campaign.

Where are the docu-dramas, more commonly known as soap operas, with a storyline about incontinence? Daytime drama is taken seriously by millions of Americans. Recently one of the most popular characters on "All My Children" had her vision saved by laser surgery, which is helping to restore and protect the eyesight of millions of diabetics. People all over the country can be made aware of medical problems and new technology through a fictional character. Producers are aware of the good they can accomplish, and these programs have very few taboos left.

The key to gain media support is to demonstrate that there is something serious to be said about incontinence and that the affliction involves a statistically significant percentage of the public—meaning *there is a market*. The editorial boards of both the print and electronic media can help by calling public attention to the problems.

The medical community should be the target of a parallel effort in the public education campaign. Doctors need better information to supply to patients—educational brochures, books, newsletters, etc. There is a measure of this going on currently, but it is not sufficient. Attention to the medical community must also include nursing homes, which need better information in counseling and handling incontinent patients. Residents of nursing homes or senior-citizen facilities are entitled to information concerning new developments that might be of help to them. Too often, entering the nursing home means minimal maintenance until death.

Another thrust of the public education campaign must be directed toward the advertising community. Those lobbying in behalf of the incontinent must aggressively press for fair and proper access to commercial time and space. This should be done through direct requests to the advertising agencies (nothing will turn them on to the need for such advertising like the recognition of potential clients) and the advertising outlets (which will be the most reluctant). Demand for access should be directed at both the paid-time commercials and the free public service opportunities. It is essential that the industry manufacturing incontinence products be heavily involved in this phase of the effort. Although its support is generally necessary, its role as prospective paid advertiser gives it a unique advantage in the thrust.

Finally, the battle must be joined at the governmental level. A comprehensive review of legislation and regulations relating to incontinence should be undertaken. Are new laws needed to ensure the rights of the incontinent against arbitrary barriers? Is some new language needed in rules regulating medical-care facilities? Do medicare and medicaid provide adequate benefits for incontinent patients?

These are a few elements necessary in the campaign to bring incontinence to the level of "public issue." They are by no means all the options. The most important element, however, is a cohesive and coordinated central strategy. To the extent that this public campaign can be coordinated through a central operation—a trade association, medical group, etc.—the effort will be more successful. The very problem today is that the issue is being presented by too many "small" voices. It now needs an identifiable authority around which the divergent interest can rally. It needs a group solely devoted to incontinence.

Based on the numbers, incontinence may be one of the greatest "hidden" afflictions of the 1980s. It deserves better treatment—medically, socially, and in our everyday human interactions.

12
Only a Beginning
Cheryle B. Gartley

At this point you are no doubt well aware that even though the topic of urinary incontinence is still taboo in America, research to solve and manage the problem is widespread and multidisciplinary.

Not long ago the first continence clinic was started in this country. The number of responses has been so great that the clinic is overwhelmed, not only by patients but also by medical professionals who hope to bring this service to their own communities. Scientists in the field of behavioral medicine at centers like Johns Hopkins University are testing biofeedback devices to help people relearn the use of the correct muscles to control incontinence. NASA technology is being harnessed and used by private enterprise to develop an external collection device that will fit the female body. Manufacturers are constantly seeking more absorbent and better-fitting garments. Machines are being developed to test incontinence products under all types of simulated conditions.

This book was written to show you in every way possible that incontinence, no matter the cause or severity, can be *managed*. People experiencing incontinence are caught up in a very intricate social and medical problem. Many doctors simply aren't prepared by their training to address the complex challenges of chronic problems. Physicians expect to cure their patients. The incontinent person find that he cannot get medical help for his incontinence even though his other medical needs are met. Doctors simply aren't prepared to address the same challenge over and over again. No wonder the incontinent person frequently slips through the cracks, finding little or no professional help!

Within these pages we hope to effect a great change, to redefine incontinence from a passively accepted disability to a challenge that can be managed and dealt with actively. Daily management is the key.

In the chapter on experiences you read how others adjusted, learned to cope, and eventually returned to useful living. The medical chapters are intended to provide you with insight into your own individual incontinence and help you to work more effectively with your doctor to manage your disability. Better medical care is at least partially the result of an informed and assertive patient.

114

Managing incontinence begins with managing your own feelings. Practicing daily all the self-help suggestions in the two chapters on emotional adjustment will bring about change. Achieving a better self-image will also improve your relationships with others. I hope by this time you can fully recognize that those who are not incontinent also have a great deal of growing to do. The chapter on relationships makes it very clear that attitudes are the real disability.

The process of changing our society begins within each of us. In light of the chapters you have just read, take a moment to examine your own attitude about the loss of urinary control.

Each of us knows cognitively that bodily functions are healthy and good, not shameful. When working properly, our bodies allow each of us a house in which our spirits, souls, personalities, emotions—everything that makes us distinctly human—can function. However, we live in a society that continually bombards us with data about the singular importance of the beauty of our bodies. But how many of us truly believe that? Do you?

The last time you were ill or had a serious crisis, was it a gorgeous woman who acted thoughtfully, or the kindly gray-haired lady next door who brought a casserole? Check out your best friend; is he handsome or is beauty in the eye of the beholder? Is he bright, fun, and supportive?

Let's all call into question what our bodies are. It's time in this society to get it straight: our bodies are our homes, to be as well maintained as possible. Individual attitudes on this topic are important because collectively they become a social attitude that then is passed on from generation to generation.

All of us, in examining and changing our own behavior, can then be in a position to contribute to changing public attitudes about incontinence. For it is, first and foremost, a *social* problem. Most of us, if we have an incontinent episode in private, find it a nuisance, but only in the company of others does incontinence suddenly seem shameful or embarrassing.

If you are incontinent, you can tell someone. Start with the dog or your favorite plant if you must, but begin to force those difficult words out of your mouth. Courage, someone once said, is grace under pressure. Talking about incontinence, learning to cope with an incontinent episode in public, coming "out of the closet"—these *do* take courage. But only for a while. Each time it gets easier.

By speaking up and learning to cope with incontinence, you will be presenting a role model for everyone who touches your life. Statistics tell us that approximately ten to twelve millions Americans are incontinent. You can readily see that your example will be affecting several people who may be quietly struggling with this problem in isolation.

Everyone who has been involved in the production of this book has his own story to tell about reaching out. Sue, who transcribed all the interviews, was telling her elderly mother about several projects she had been working on, but the one her mother seemed intent on hearing more about was the incontinence book. Sue suddenly realized what was happening and asked her mother directly if she were experiencing incontinence. Thus by a chance phone conversation an entire family's puzzlement as to why their mother hadn't made her usual Christmas visit was solved. Reach out, and tell somebody!

If you are not incontinent, this is still your challenge. Reread closely Chapters 2 and 3 of this book and you will see once again how important your attitudes about incontinence also are. Take a minute to think carefully about what you would do and how you would like to be treated if you were experiencing incontinence. An example of how badly we all need sensitizing to the plight of incontinent people can be seen in the following story.

In 1983 a newsletter containing information for ambulatory and wheel-chair persons with urinary incontinence had the following statement tucked in one corner: "The members of ———— are not necessarily incontinent; however, they are all genuinely interested in helping others." Think back to the last time someone rang your doorbell to ask for a donation to the American Cancer Society or some other worthy cause. Did that person begin by telling you that he himself didn't have the disease but was genuinely interested in helping others? The stigma surrounding urinary incontinence in our society is so deep that well-meaning people don't realize the impact of their words on the incontinent.

In fact, I understand the rationale for such statements. My reasoning was similar several months ago when this project started. I then had absolutely no intention of participating in it personally. My role was to be the editor. Then Jill insisted on interviewing me. And then everyone connected with the book insisted on not granting me anonymity. And finally my dear friend Martha wrote the preface that shoved me completely out of the closet and slammed the door forever behind me. (Thank you, Mat.) The point of no return has now been reached. I am affected by incontinence and initially did everything you've just learned you are not supposed to do. I withdrew to my home, rejected my friends, told no one, and of course became isolated and depressed. I was thirty and life had abruptly stopped.

But a few friends, persistent friends, would not let me withdraw, and they finally unraveled the truth. A chance remark by one of them became a turning point. He simply wondered in frustration what they were doing for the women they intended to put into space. One day, on impulse, I decided to find out. Although transferred through half the staff at NASA, my call finally landed at the right desk. Not, however, before the phone bill equaled the mortgage payment that month.

Through my growing friendships with the people at NASA and Research Triangle Institute and others already working on the challenge of incontinence, I learned many things. I also read everything from medical textbooks to European studies. Most important, I discovered, to my surprise, that I wasn't alone—the estimates were into the millions. Depression gave way to knowledge and knowledge to anger, and that anger, somewhat tempered, birthed this book and the Simon Foundation.

In 1983 several dedicated professionals joined with me to found this organization. As we go to press, the Simon Foundation is still in its embryonic stage, but we are growing by leaps and bounds as the word reaches out. In addition to *Managing Incontinence*, we publish a quarterly newsletter, have a study in progress about emotional adjustment to incontinence, and expect to release a docu-drama film in the next few months.

The tip of the iceberg has been sighted, but its depth remains unmeasured, and there is much to do. When the Simon Foundation is built, we will have an 800 WATS line to answer questions, distribute product literature, and encourage those who are beginning to seek to manage their incontinence. One movie will become a series. There will be a second edition of *Managing Incontinence*, for already we know that this is far from all there is to say; topics such as enuresis and fecal incontinence remain to be explored.

Programs for the medical professions are planned. We will speak out about restrictions on advertising and detrimental policies of our government bodies. First and foremost, however, will always be communication with people who are struggling daily with the problem of incontinence.

Recently a man wrote to us: "I want to thank you for mailing the 'Informer' [Simon Foundation newsletter] to us. It has given my wife new hope. The problem is caused by Parkinson's disease and life has been severe since she was stricken, but your publication has given us hope for the future."

The overall message of this book is HOPE.

A Personal Note from the Editor

Eventually, wherever I speak someone will ask me what Simon stands for. It is a question I love to answer and this book would not be complete without your knowing too.

Simon was my grandfather, and although in many ways an ordinary man, he was very special. He had a belief that was central to his life. He believed that in this country anything was possible. Crawling across the border of his own beloved country, Latvia, at risk to his life, he made his way to this country with only the shirt on his back. A tailor by trade, he opened a small business, which supported his wife and four children, and which eventually enabled him to purchase even an automobile.

He died when I was twenty-one, but the tapes of our conversations still play in my memory. When I got my first pair of real shoes, Capizzio's no less, grandpa said, "In this country, they look great on you." In Italy would they have looked terrible? When I became a fairly proficient clarinetist and grandfather would hear my newest piece, he would respond, "In this country, you will make a terrific professional musician." Anywhere else I would have sounded like an amateur, no doubt. When the tragedy of braces on my teeth befell me at age eighteen, grandpa thought that they were beautiful, because, of course, where else but in America could the dentists perform such miracles!

Once, and only once, in the rebellious teenage years did I contradict him. I remember telling him in an outburst that in this country only girls that were beautiful got to be cheerleaders, that in this country only the "rich" people got dates to the boatclub parties, and, furthermore, that in this country one of my friends, who happened to be black, couldn't get a haircut in any barbershop in our town. By that time he had been in America for over half a century, so he knew that killing granddaughters here, even teenage ones, was a crime. After he stopped breathing heavily, and the red left his face, he said, "In this country, everything can be changed."

The Simon Foundation is named after this man, to challenge everyone who believes as he did—those who see a wrong and believe it can be made right—and to motivate a granddaughter.

Acknowledgments

It would take many pages to recognize here all who have helped, inspired, educated, and influenced me. Yet a few stand out because I remember a kind word, an attitude, or an action, perhaps ever so slight, that made the difference in how my life was shaped. For there remain unexplored forces in the universe—both for the light and the dark. In part this book was written for and because of the following people:

BILL GARTLEY— My husband, whose acceptance of this problem is so thorough I'm not quite sure if he yet fully understands why the world is not ready for this book to be called "Free to Pee." He believed in me for a long time.

CHRISTINE GASSER—My friend since kindergarten, to whom it never occurred I might not be able to leap from barn lofts. She always stands ready to give me the shirt off her back, and indeed has.

STAN BRANDON, M.D.—The orthopedist who kept fighting to save my leg when no one else would. If we could clone the whole medical profession after him, the industry built on malpractice insurance would be out of business tomorrow. And for BARBARA his wife, who treated me like a sister.

MARTHA TEICHNER—Despite her obvious success in a tough field, she always thought that the work I did from my kitchen table was just as important. I have heard from her from far corners of the world, and her encouragement never faltered.

BARRY ULLMAN—Who never cared what awful things he put on my feet and had the nerve to call shoes, as long as I walked without pain. He healed a leg that most of medicine deemed beyond hope.

JOHN HUMPAL—Who finally, and with great patience and long hours of conversation, convinced me we all have defects and in a sense armed me with the strength to be myself.

RON ROZENSKY—My shrink, who has walked in a million different moccasins with great empathy and comes away so beautifully whole.

JEAN CAVANAUGH, M.D.—My physician. She raises a family, practices medicine, and still returns telephone calls within twenty minutes when you are ill. She is friend, healer, and advocate.

THE BEAST—My husband's IBM PC. A salute to all the brainpower that made it possible, for with it man can extend himself to the edges of the universe.

SIMON BLUMBERG—My grandfather, who came to this country with only the clothes on his back and for whom the Simon Foundation is named. He thought in America all things were possible.

LARRY P. HORIST—Who ordered me to write this book. He gave me ideas and training freely, and taught me that the greatest power in the world is an idea for good . . . made into a reality.

NAN AND MILLER SLAUGHTER—Who between them have seen plenty of the dark side of life and choose light. They lead the way by example. I love them both.

LUCILLE BLUMBERG—My mother. The greatest thing you can say about a person is he did the best he could. She taught me that "nothing in the world can take the place of persistence. Talent will not; nothing is more common than unsuccessful men with talent. Genius will not; unrewarded genius is almost a proverb. Education alone will not; the world is full of educated derelicts. Persistence and determination alone are omnipotent." She did the best she could.

HERMAN BLUMBERG—My father, who spent many a summer night teaching a differently abled girl who wanted to play softball with the boys, that if she got close enough to the ball to touch it, there was no excuse acceptable if she dropped it. It has become a life rule: if you get close enough to have a chance at something, go for it. In a way, the way my father looked at life, plus that childhood lesson learned so well, explains better than anything else, how this book came about.

WAYNE JARVIS—Our best man, who stashed champagne in our suitcase when none of us could afford it, and gives continuity to my life now, when I need it most.

RON AND JILL BALSON—From time to time they've both given me their professional talents, but what is most important in my life is that they have given to me themselves.

JANE ALVARO—Who could teach a whole world how to enjoy life. Her sunshine and faith in this idea light up my life.

KATE JETER—Who has done more than anyone else I have met to fight for human dignity for all mankind. Her energy reaches out to touch all she meets, and her encouragement has been very special to me.

DAVID ZEHREN, who kicked me into coming out of the closet. DORIS HOWELL, whose sincere encouragement means more to me than she'll ever know. LINDA BLUMBERG, who gave me a chance when no one else would. JOHN KANE, deep thanks for spending some time on me; it will be passed on to others. DR. PAUL BRAND, whose long hours of research and training trained others. TERI CAMPBELL and KEN STREMMING, who introduced me to the universe. BILL GRAMLEY, BARBARA EDWARDS JOHNSON, and MARY JANE RADTKE, who got me through college. LORETTA HOLM KUMMER and DIANE

LEMPKE, who never left me in spirit. BARB MORRIS, who often makes sense for me of a senseless world. ADRIENE MEISEL, with whom I can pick up the phone tomorrow and it will be like yesterday. And DAN HALES, his competency and integrity are an ever present reminder of what to reach for in all one's interactions.

CHUCK STOCKING, FRAN BOUDA, MATTS DORING, BILL DAVIDSON . . . newfound friends in the incontinence manufacturing industry, men who do more than their jobs. All of corporate America should be like these.

RICHARD WHEELER—the editor's editor, encourager, and friend.

JAMESON CAMPAIGNE, JR—The editor's publisher, whose hard business approach disguises a great deal of softness and produces the money to take a gamble on a groundbreaking book like this. Thanks.

SAM SCHILLER—A fine designer who organized, needled, and laughed us through this project.

If we succeed in this task, it is because pieces of us all were mixed together and from this synergism came forces for good.

Contributors

The people who wrote this book are as varied as the problem itself. Some wrote from their kitchen tables, with children and pets too constant companions. Others wrote from offices at prestigious universities and hospitals. One wrote from a hotel in Damascus. They all had a common denominator, however: the wish to improve life for you and your family.

LARRY P. HORIST—L. P. Horist is chairman of L. P. Horist and Associates, Inc., a government relations and public-affairs firm. Unlike traditional public relations firms, LPH&A's main thrust is to mold opinion on public issues and to influence directly the implementation of public policy. His clients include Fortune 500 companies, national and state associations, issue-oriented groups, and major political candidates. Mr. Horist frequently appears on radio and television talk shows as a public policy expert. He has lectured on college and university campuses, including Institute of Politics of the John F. Kennedy School of Government at Harvard.

HENRY HOLDEN—Actor and comedian. Henry has performed in a variety of regional and off-Broadway plays, in TV's "Kojak," and in the films *An Unmarried Woman*, *Chapter Two*, and *Seventh Avenue*. He is a graduate of C. W. Post College on Long Island and has studied acting under Lee Strasberg. Holden is the first chairman of the committee for performers with disabilities of the Screen Actors Guild. He lectures on college campuses through the country on "Attitudes Are the Real Disability." "Real People" recently focused on Holden's special brand of humor.

JOHN J. HUMPAL, PH.D.—Professor of business policy and behavioral science at the University of Chicago Graduate School of Business. John was a Standard Oil of Indiana Fellow and a National Defense Education Act Scholar. His dissertation was awarded the 1973 Creative Talents Prize by the American Institute for Research. He consults extensively and represents the University of Chicago in national and international management seminars. John is also on the Governing Board of the Simon Foundation.

CHERYLE B. GARTLEY—Founder and president of the Simon Foundation. Cheryle is currently an M.B.A. candidate at the University of Chicago. She is listed in the 1978 edition of *Outstanding Young Women of America*. She is a cofounder of Veterans Day in Evanston and a founding board member of Seniors Actions Services, Inc. Cheryle also lectures and writes on various topics concerning spina bifida.

JEAN CAVANAUGH, M.D.—Assistant Professor, Clinical, Rehabilitation Medicine, Northwestern University Medical School. Jean is an attending staff physician at Evanston-Glenbrook Hospitals. She is a board member of the Evanston Safety Education Center, and is active in several other community organizations, including: Illinois Child Passenger Safety Association, Utilization Review Committee of the Evanston Visiting Nurse Association, and Professional Advisory Board of the Evanston Visiting Nurse Association. She is also a founding member of the Advisory Board of the Simon Foundation.

JANE ALVARO—Prospect research coordinator, Chicago Symphony Orchestra. Jane has a B.S. in psychology from College of the Holy Cross in Worcester, Massachusetts. She has had a lifelong interest in music, and studied abroad her junior year in Austria. Jane is a fundraising consultant for the Simon Foundation.

STEVEN M. TOVIAN, PH.D.—Clinical psychologist and director of Psychodiagnostic Evaluation and Testing Services, Department of Psychiatry, Evanston Hospital; director of Psychosocial Counseling Services, Kellogg Cancer Care Center, Evanston Hospital; associate professor, Northwestern University Medical School, Department of Psychiatry, Division of Psychology. Steve is a member of the Psychosocial Advisory Board, Illinois Cancer Council; chairman of the Thanatology Committee, Evanston Hospital; and a founding member of the Advisory Board of the Simon Foundation.

RONALD H. ROZENSKY, PH.D.—Assistant chairman for research and evaluation, Department of Psychiatry, Evanston Hospital; associate clinical professor of psychiatry and behavioral science, Northwestern University Medical School; associate professor of psychology, Department of Psychology, Northwestern University; member Cancer Care Advisory Board, Evanston Hospital. Ron is also a clinical psychologist whose major research interest is psychosocial factors in a therapeutic milieu, self-control issues, and emotional response to illness. Ron is in private practice in Evanston, Illinois.

WILLIAM A. GARTLEY—Independent computer applications consultant. Bill is an expert both in solving business problems and in simplifying business operations through computer applications. Much of his professional work involves gathering information from diverse sources and translating that information into nontechnical language so that the users can better understand and manage their computers. He has a B.S. in biology/chemistry, did postgraduate work in mathematics and computer science at Northwestern University, and holds an M.B.A. in finance from the University of Chicago.

ROSEMARIE B. KING, R.N., M.S.—Assistant director of nursing, Rehabilitation Institute of Chicago. Rosemarie is the chairman of the Sexuality Committee at the institute. She lectures widely on sexuality, incontinence, and other topics related to disabilities. Incontinence has long been an area of interest for her. She is coauthor of an award-winning slide-tape educational program for nurses on urinary incontinence and its management. Rosemarie recently published a chapter titled "Assessment and Management of Soft Tissue Pressure" in the McGraw-Hill publication *Comprehensive Rehabilitative Nursing.*

WILLIAM E. KAPLAN, M.D.—Director of neurologic urology, Children's Memorial Hospital, Chicago, and assistant professor of urology, Northwestern University. Bill is a leading advocate of the use of clean intermittent catheterization for children with spina bifida. He also is a leader in promoting artificial sphincter implantation for children. Bill gives of his time freely, sitting on the advisory boards of many associations and foundations, including the Spina Bifida Association, the Urologic Council of the Kidney Foundation, the Advisory Council for Independent Living and Rehabilitation, and the Simon Foundation.

KATHERINE JETER, Ed.D., E.T.—Katherine is one of the pioneers of enterostomal therapy. She recently published *These Special Children: The Ostomy Book for Parents and Children with Colostomies, Ileostomies, and Urostomies.* Katherine lectures internationally on the topic of incontinence. She is on the Professional Advisory Board of the United Ostomy Association, the Governing Board of the Simon Foundation, and founder of HIP (Help for Incontinent People), Union, S.C.

ALISON BACH GOOD—Illustrator. Ms. Good brings to her artwork a broad background of experience. A native of Rochester, Minnesota, she earned a B.A. from Colorado Women's College in Denver, and did graduate work at the University of Saskatchewan School of Medicine and at the University of Minnesota College of Education. Ms. Good has taught studio art and biology at the junior and senior high school level, and has worked as a commercial artist. As a member of the auxiliary of the Evanston-Glenbrook Hospitals, she coordinated the development of a closed-circuit TV channel for patient education. She is coordinator for the National High School Institute at Northwestern University and freelances as a medical illustrator. Ms. Good, her husband, and two children live in Wilmette, Illinois.

JILL BALSON, M.A.—Jill has an undergraduate degree in education from the University of Illinois and a masters in guidance and counseling from Loyola University in Chicago. She taught primary grades for four years in the Chicago public schools and has long been interested in developmental psychology. The focus of her master's thesis was high school underachievement. Jill, her husband, and three children live in Highland Park, Illinois.

MARTHA A. TEICHNER—Martha is a correspondent for CBS News, based since April 1, 1984, in Dallas. In her previous postings with the network, first in Atlanta, then in London, she traveled extensively, covering stories in Latin America, Europe, and the Middle East. In 1980 she won the John F. Kennedy Journalism Award for the radio documentary "The Freedom Flotilla," on the Cuban boatlift. Before joining CBS in 1977 Miss Teichner was a reporter for television stations in Chicago, Miami, and Grand Rapids and before that for a radio station in Grand Rapids. She is a 1969 Wellesley College graduate with a degree in economics and attended the University of Chicago Graduate School of Business. She has been a member of the Advisory Board of the Simon Foundation since its inception.

Appendix 1

The following appendix was produced from information supplied by manufacturers that the author contacted. It is not a complete list of all products available. Many manufacturers have additional products and there are manufacturers that have not been included. To be included in this list is not a recommendation or guarantee nor is any liability implied or assumed by the author.

Please be aware that specifications and products may change. It is best to consult your doctor or pharmacist or the manufacturer before purchasing. Most are available without a prescription. It is best to buy minimum quantities at first to be sure that the product meets the required need.

People familiar with incontinence have found that there is no real uniformity of terms or classification of products. The author also faced this problem and for the sake of expediency has ordered the appendix alphabetically by manufacturer's and distributor's name. Each product, however, is classified by general purpose(s) or function(s).

MANUFACTURER:	**Aegis Medical, Inc.**
PRODUCT NAME:	**Avatar™ 2000 Bowel Evacuation System (Hospital, Institutional Use)** **Avatar™ Personal Bowel Care System (Home Use)**
USE:	**For people who experience episodic or chronic bowel dysfunction or management. Safe for everyday use.**
DESCRIPTION:	The Avatar system incorporates a unique approach to bowel evacuation and operates on a new principle called PIEE, Pulsed Irrigation For Enhanced Evacuation.
Benefits:	AVATAR eliminates involuntary bowel movements, removes impactions which can cause constipation, eliminates the need for laxatives and suppositories, AND greatly reduces bowel program time.
Applications:	Chronic constipation, incontinence, spinal cord injury, spina bifida, multiple sclerosis, outpatient use, neuromuscular disease, impaction removal, surgery preparation, GI procedures.
PACKAGING:	Each treatment uses an AvaPak™ Individual Sanitary Bowel Treatment Pak, which are single use components packaged 16 per case, that ensure a clean and safe procedure.
CONTACT:	Aegis Medical's Personal Care Advisors Aegis Medical, Inc. 370 17th Street, Suite 700 Denver, Colorado 80202 Telephone: 303-592-2050 1-800-232-9919

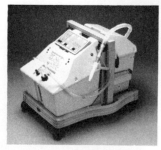

Avatar Personal Bowel Care System
(Home Use)

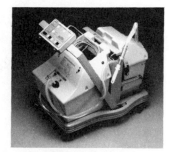

Avatar 2000 Bowel Evacuation System
(Hospital Use)

MANUFACTURER:	**American Medical Systems, Inc.**
PRODUCT NAME:	**AMS Sphincter 800™ Urinary Prosthesis**
USE:	**A surgically implantable device designed to control the leakage of urine from the body.**
DESCRIPTION:	The AMS Sphincter 800™ is designed to mimic the natural process of urinary control and urination. Like the body's natural sphincter, the AMS Sphincter 800 causes the urethra to close; this makes it possible for the bladder to store urine. To urinate, the patient opens the urethra by squeezing the device's pump. After urination, the device automatically recloses the urethra and continence is restored.
AVAILABILITY:	Urologists have implanted artificial urinary sphincters in more than 5,000 men and women, boys and girls. Some leading causes of urinary incontinence for those already implanted have been, among men, radical prostatectomy and transurethral resection; among children, myelomeningocele; and, among women, severe stress incontinence.
CONTACT:	(For information and a list of urologists working with artificial urinary sphincters) American Medical Systems Department SF P.O. Box 9 Minneapolis, MN 55440 Phone: 1-800/328-3881 (in Minnesota, 612/933-4666).

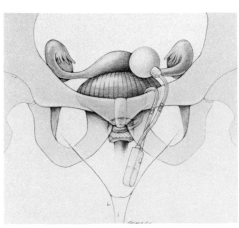

The AMS Sphincter 800™ Urinary Prosthesis implanted within the body.

MANUFACTURER:	**Biotechnologies, Inc.**
PRODUCT NAME:	**PerryMeter™ Incontinence Treatment Systems**
USE:	**Any type of urinary or fecal incontinence**
DESCRIPTION:	This instrument allows monitoring and rehabilitation of pelvic floor muscles while patient remains fully clothed. A light display on the EMG Biofeedback device provides visual indication of muscle activity, allowing most patients to learn to strengthen their own sphincters for complete control without surgery or drugs. Available for purchase, although usually rented for one or two month's use at home. (No electrical stimulation is needed.)
ALSO AVAILABLE:	Several models, styles and sizes are available. Also, computerized muscle diagnostic and training systems, for the therapist's office, provide printed reports and graphic video biofeedback.
CONTACT:	PerryMeter™ Systems Division Biotechnologies, Inc. P.O. Box 256 Bryn Mawr, PA 19010 Telephone: 800-537-3779 or 215-525-8778

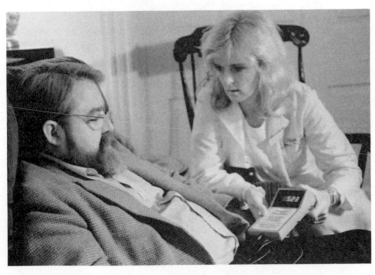

Most patients learn to strengthen their sphincter muscles in six to eight weeks of daily at-home practice.

MANUFACTURER:	**Chattem, Inc.**
PRODUCT NAME:	**NULLO deodorant tablets**
USE:	**For controlling odor due to urinary incontinence, fecal incontinence, colostomy and ileostomy.**
DESCRIPTION:	Each tablet contains 33.3 mg. of chlorophyllin copper complex which clinical studies have reported consistent results in controlling body odors due to the above conditions. In June, 1985, following consideration of a report from the Advisory Review Panel, the Food and Drug Administration issued a proposed final ruling that specifically identifies chlorophyllin copper complex as being safe and effective, taken orally, in reducing urinary and fecal odors related to incontinence and for odor due to colostomies and ileostomies.
DOSAGE:	Adults twelve years of age and older, swallow one or two tablets three times a day, depending on severity of odor, until odor is eliminated (from two to ten days). Then take one tablet three times a day or as needed to control odor. For children under twelve years of age, consult a physician.
PACKAGING:	NULLO deodorant tablets come in bottles containing 30, 60 and 135 tablets.
AVAILABILITY:	Available without a prescription at medical supply houses, drugstores, pharmacies and through incontinence and ostomy supply mail order houses.
ALSO AVAILABLE:	Pamphlet on *Incontinence* covering prevalence, types, causes, treatment options and daily management. Pamphlet on NULLO deodorant tablets giving background, dosage, clinical data and other information. NULLO product samples.
CONTACT:	Chattem, Inc., Att: Professional Services 1715 W. 38th Street, Chattanooga, TN 37409 1-800-366-6833

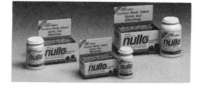

MANUFACTURER:	**Hollister Incorporated**
PRODUCT NAME:	**Hollister® Female Urinary Incontinence System**
USE:	**For ambulatory or non-ambulatory women with bladder control problems related to stress, urge or overflow incontinence.**
DESCRIPTION:	Female Urinary Incontinence System features Female Urinary Device which encompasses the urethral meatus with a form-fitting pericup. The device acts as a conduit, funneling urine away from the body, through flexible Extension Tubing and into a Urinary Thigh Bag. A combination of the woman's anatomy and a pair of support pants holds the device in place **without** the use of adhesives. Leg Bag Straps, Disposable Sizing Device, Cleansing Tablets and Silicone Lubricant complete the System.
PACKAGING:	System components, excluding the device which must be sized by a professional, are available in a Starter Kit. The Female Urinary Device is sold separately and comes with two Extension Tube Assemblies. System components may also be purchased separately.

ALSO AVAILABLE:	Hollister Incorporated offers a complete line of incontinence products for men and women.
	    Male Urinary Collection System:
	      Self-Adhesive Urinary External Catheter (4 sizes)
	      Self-Adhesive Urinary External Catheter with Removable Tip for Intermittent Catherization (2 sizes)
	      Urinary Leg Bag, Vented Urinary Leg Bag (2 sizes)
	    Retracted Penis Pouch, Female Urinary Pouch
	    Drainable Fecal Incontinence Collector (2 sizes)
	    Leg Bag Straps (3 sizes), Extension Tubing

CONTACT:	Hollister Incorporated 2000 Hollister Drive Libertyville, Illinois 60048 Phone toll-free: in Illinois 1-800-942-1141 in the US 1-800-323-4060, in Canada 1-800-263-7400

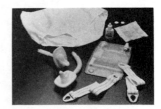

COMPANY:	**Home Delivery Incontinent Supplies Co. (HDIS)**
PRODUCTS:	**Mail order delivery of all major absorbent product lines, skin care items, and catheters, including: DEPEND, ATTENDS, TRANQUILITY, SURETYS, SERENITY, PROMISE, and many other brands.**
DESCRIPTION:	HDIS offers shop-at-home *convenience* and *privacy* for people with bladder control needs. Our caring, professional staff will assist you in choosing the right product for your needs. Our *fast, doorstep delivery* by UPS means you'll receive your order in just 1-5 days. All orders are sent in discreet *unmarked boxes.* And, our low "buy-by-the-case" prices usually mean big *savings!*
ALSO AVAILABLE:	Free Catalog and free product samples
CONTACT:	HDIS P.O. Box 52039 St. Louis, MO 63136 Call Toll Free: 1-800-538-1036

BLADDER CONTROL HELP ...
JUST A PHONE CALL AWAY!

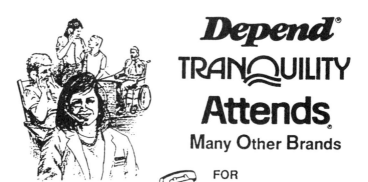

Depend®

TRANQUILITY

Attends®

Many Other Brands

FOR INFO CALL **1-800-538-1036**

MANUFACTURER:	**Johnson & Johnson**
PRODUCT NAME:	**SERENITY® Guards**
USE:	**For moderate and severe female urinary incontinence**
DESCRIPTION:	The compact and discreet SERENITY® Guards gives you the protection you need—right where you need it most. That's because SERENITY® contains a unique superabsorbent system that traps liquid quickly and effectively. A fine powder locks this liquid into a gel that can't leak.
	SERENITY® Guards are contoured to fit a woman's natural shape for better protection against leakage. Each guard has a soft, waterproof outer lining and a smooth top layer that keeps wetness away from the skin.
PACKAGING:	Individually folded and wrapped in 3 absorbencies: Light (14 guards/box), Regular (12 or 36 guards/box), and Super (10 or 30 guards/box).
CONTACT:	Toll-free number 1-800-962-1129 ext. 304 8:00 a.m. to 5:00 p.m. Eastern
	or write to: Johnson & Johnson P.O. Box 5234 Clifton, New Jersey 07015

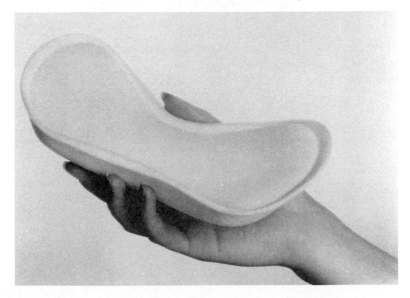

MANUFACTURER:	**Kendall-Futuro**
PRODUCT NAME:	**Curity® Disposable Contoured Briefs**
USE:	**For maximum bladder and bowel control protection**

DESCRIPTION:

- Patented Leak-Pruf Stripes™ trap fluid and inhibit leakage
- Ultra-absorbent fluff filler absorbs over 14 times its own weight in moisture
- Waterproof outer layer provides added security
- Wetness Indicator on outside poly changes color when garment is wet—ideal for caretakers
- Four refastenable tape tabs provide a customized fit—time after time
- Flexible, elastic leg gathers keep brief comfortably snug and secure

PACKAGING: Available in Small, Medium, and Large in 10-count poly bags

ALSO AVAILABLE: Disposable Underpads, Brief Liners, Waterproof Sheeting, Reusable Incontinence Pants, Free Consumer Booklet

CONTACT: The Kendall-Futuro Company,
Curity® Bladder Control Products
5801 Mariemont Ave.
Cincinnati, OH 45227
1-800-543-4452 (Ohio residents call 1-800-686-3400)

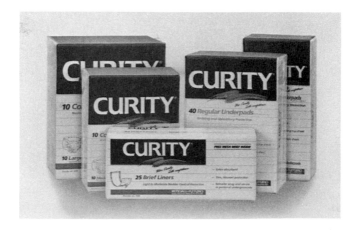

MANUFACTURER:	**Kimberly-Clark Corporation**
PRODUCT NAME:	**DEPEND® Absorbent Products**
USE:	**For light, moderate to complete loss of bladder control.**

DESCRIPTION: Available in four distinct product forms, each designed to address a specific incontinence need.

Shields—cup shape conforms to the body for discreetness and comfort. (Available in regular and extra absorbencies)

Undergarments—design is virtually undetectable under clothing with open sides for comfort and freedom of movement—ideal for even the most active people. (Available in regular and extra absorbencies)

Fitted Briefs—elastic at the waist and legs and six refastenable tapes provide maximum protection for heavy to complete loss of bladder control. (Available in regular and large sizes)

Underpads—special layers of absorbent materials protect bed, chair, and other surfaces. (Available in bed and chair sizes)

PACKAGING: Available in trial, regular, convenience, and thrifty packs

CONTACT: Kimberly-Clark Corporation
P.O. Box 2002
Neenah, WI 54956-9002

For more information on DEPEND absorbent products or to obtain a free sample, call:
In Wisconsin 1-800-242-6463
Outside Wisconsin 1-800-558-6423

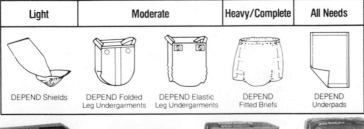

Light	Moderate		Heavy/Complete	All Needs
DEPEND Shields	DEPEND Folded Leg Undergarments	DEPEND Elastic Leg Undergarments	DEPEND Fitted Briefs	DEPEND Underpads

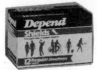

MANUFACTURER:	**Med-I-Pant Inc.**
PRODUCT NAME:	**Med-I-Brief, Med-I-Liner & Med-I-Pad**
USE:	**For all levels of incontinence**
DESCRIPTION:	<u>Med-I-Brief</u> is designed for the ambulatory. Fully adjustable leak-proof design. Super absorbant, naturally soft and simple to use. <u>Med-I-Liner</u> provides economical and discreet protection for light to medium incontinence. <u>Med-I-Pad</u> for ultimate protection in bed. A single unit replacement for plastic sheets, draw sheets and all disposable products.
	<u>Note:</u> All MED-I-PANT products are machine washable and extra-long lasting.
PACKAGING:	Individually or in bulk
ALSO AVAILABLE:	Catalogue and In-Service Information
CONTACT:	MED-I-PANT INC.
	4100 Parthenais Street
	Montreal, Quebec H2K-3T9
	514/522-1224

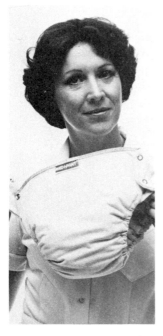 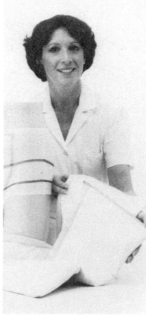 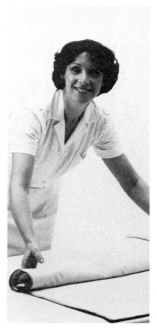

COMPANY:	**Principle Business Enterprises, Inc.**

PRODUCTS:	**Tranquility**

DESCRIPTION:

Light or stress— TrimShields have adhesive strips which fit into the wearer's own underwear. The patented construction features a special gel-forming material which locks urine in securely. There is virtually no squeeze-out.

Moderate—The brief and high capacity pad system offers the ultimate protection for ambulatory users. The washable brief has a moisture proof lining and two loops to hold the pad securely. It has the same gel-forming material as the TrimShields.

Heavy—The SlimLine disposable underpant comes in four sizes: youth, small, medium and large. The special "Peach Mat Guarantee" assures the wearer of excellent dryness, protects against skin irritation, and significantly reduces odor. The underpant is very discreet and trim-fitting with no excess bulk. It can be worn under regular clothing.

PACKAGING:

TrimShields—regular-12 per box, super-10 per box
Briefs—1 per box
Starter kit—1 brief and 3 pads per box
High Capacity Pads—25 per box or 10 per box
SlimLine—youth-10 per box, small-10 per box, medium-8 per box, large-8 per box

HOW AVAILABLE:

Home health care stores and mail order catalogs. The product is not available directly from the company.

CONTACT:

Principle Business Enterprises, Inc.
Pine Lake Industrial Park
Dunbridge, OH 43414

For additional information, the company has a toll-free network at 1-800-843-3385 or 1-800-843-2365 (in Ohio).

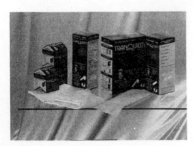
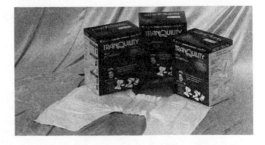

MANUFACTURER:	**Procter & Gamble**
PRODUCT NAME:	**Attends Disposable Briefs**
USE:	**For Major Bladder Control Problems**
DESCRIPTION:	Disposable Briefs that help provide reliable protection from leakage and odor. Unique soft lining helps keep skin dry. Heavy-duty inner padding soaks up many times its weight in moisture. Waterproof outer layer helps protect against leakage and odor. One-step re-fastenable tapes are easy to use and let you adjust the brief fit. Flexible self-adjusting leg gathers. Wetness indicator turns from yellow to blue to show when the Brief is wet.
PACKAGING:	Available in sizes Small, Medium, and Large in: 12-count poly bags; 10-count cartons; and in bulk—Small (96 Briefs), Medium (96 Briefs), and Large (48 Briefs).
CONTACT:	Procter & Gamble P.O. Box 599 Cincinnati, OH 45201 Also available through Surgical Supply Stores and Drug Stores.
TELEPHONE:	Continental U.S. 1-800-543-0480 (Ohio Residents call 1-800-582-0490)

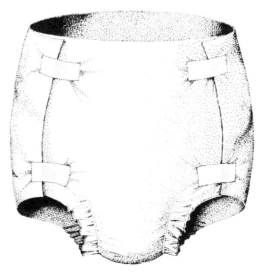

MANUFACTURER:	**Scott Health Care Products** **A Business Unit of Scott Paper Company**
PRODUCT NAME:	**Promise® Pads and Pants**
USE:	**For the full range of incontinence**
DESCRIPTION:	A unique, two-piece system of disposable, highly absorbent pads and lightweight, washable mesh pants. Promise offers superior protection and comfort because it's designed to fit and feel like real clothes. Available in a full range of pant sizes to fit the body and pad protection levels to fit the problem.
PACKAGING:	Pads are available in Light, Standard, Extra Absorbent and Nighttime protection levels. Pants come in small, medium, large and extra large and are available in packages of two or bulk pack.
CONTACT:	For complete information: Scott Health Care Products Scott Plaza I Philadelphia, PA 19113 Sales Office 1-800-992-9939 Consumer Information: 1-800-TEL-SCOT

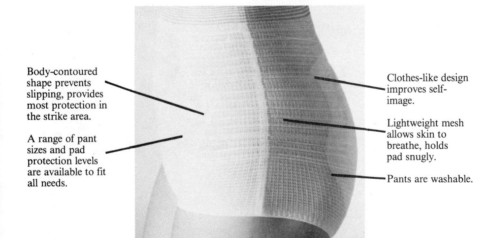

Body-contoured shape prevents slipping, provides most protection in the strike area.

A range of pant sizes and pad protection levels are available to fit all needs.

Clothes-like design improves self-image.

Lightweight mesh allows skin to breathe, holds pad snugly.

Pants are washable.

MANUFACTURER:	**Sherwood Medical**
PRODUCT NAME:	**Uri-Drain® Male Urinary Control System**
USE:	**A total system for incontinent males**
DESCRIPTION:	Individually bagged catheters in three sizes, with either foam straps or two-sided adhesive tapes and skin prep, are combined with reusable leg bags. Standard bags come in two sizes, a deluxe model in three sizes. All are made of cotton-flocked vinyl for extra comfort. Clear anti-kink extension tubing to connect catheter to leg bag also available.
ALSO AVAILABLE:	Sherwood Medical also manufactures the Texas Catheter® Brand of External Catheters.
CONTACT:	Sherwood Medical 1831 Olive Street St. Louis, MO 63103 Telephone: 1-800-527-1073

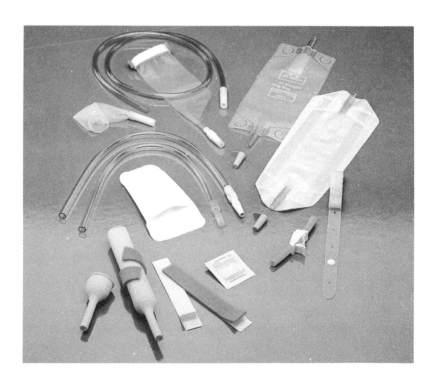

Appendix 2

Please help us by taking a moment to fill out the following questionnaire and return it to:

The Simon Foundation
Box 815
Wilmette, Illinois 60091

I purchased this book

☐ By mail direct from the publisher
☐ As a premium offer from an incontinence product manufacturer
☐ At a bookstore
☐ It was a gift from:

    ☐ friend
    ☐ spouse
    ☐ children
    ☐ other _____

Questions for those who are incontinent:

1. How long have you been incontinent? _____

2. Do you know the reason for your incontinence? _____
   If so, what causes your incontinence? _____
_____

3. Have you discussed your condition with your doctor? _____
   If so, how helpful did you find him or her?

    ☐ very, took a great deal of time exploring the topic
    ☐ somewhat, but we found no answers
    ☐ not helpful, he/she did not want to talk about incontinence

Cut along here

4. How do you manage your incontinence currently?

☐ By a surgical intervention
☐ Artificial sphincter
☐ Drug therapy
☐ Indwelling catheter
☐ External catheter
☐ Incontinence products
☐ Other _____

5. Do you feel your incontinence is managed well enough to live normally? _____ If no, please explain. _____
_____
_____

6. Do those close to you—family, friends—know that you have problems with continence? (Please tell us as much as you can about this—how these people react, how comfortable you are in telling others, etc.) ___
_____
_____

7. What needs do you have concerning this disability which are currently NOT being met? _____
_____
_____

Cut here

☐ I would like to receive the Simon Foundation's quarterly newsletter. (It is not necessary to fill in your name unless you would like to receive the newsletter.) Please send a copy of *The Informer* to:

Name _____

Street _____

City, State, Zip Code _____

The Simon Foundation
Box 815
Wilmette, Illinois 60091